Animal Care & Nursing

Physical examination

A veterinarian is responsible for supervising the veterinary technician. This includes overseeing the technician's collection of information regarding a patient's anesthesia risk factors. This information will be used to promote a comprehensive anesthesia plan. The anesthesia plan should be strictly adhered to during the performance of any procedure. Further, it should be used to check the status of a patient's recovery following the administration of anesthesia. Medical record documentation should bear out adherence to the anesthesia plan. To this end, there should be an authentication process applied for all medical record entries.

The technician is responsible for consulting with and keeping the veterinarian informed of any irregularities or unexpected situations and occurrences. The physical exam of the patient is beneficial in obtaining information about any health concerns that have not previously been addressed by a medical professional. This physical examination is the first step in assessing the patient's overall health. The technician should adhere to a preset, standard routine regarding the physical examination. This will help ensure a more complete and uniform examination. The routine also prompts the technician to adhere to important portions of the exam which may easily be overlooked when a less consistent routine is used. Each body system requires a thorough perusal in a comprehensive examination.

Skin and coat

There are a number of potential issues associated with the condition of an animal's skin and coat. Therefore, the technician should be careful to note whether or not the animal's skin and/or coat has a healthy shine to it. A dull coat may indicate that the skin is dry, and may ultimately contribute to a condition known as alopecia. Alopecia is the loss of hair or the persistent absence of hair from the body. In some animals, this can be aggravated by excessive scratching and ultimate injury to itchy, dry skin.

The skin's elasticity or turgor (i.e., hydrated plumpness) should also be examined. This evaluation can help detect problems associated with dehydration. Skin that is poorly hydrated usually does not exhibit proper flexibility, and thus will not snap back into place when pulled outward. Instead, the skin is slow to go back into place. The skin at the thoracolumbar region in particular should be pulled upon to determine if the skin can be described as properly or poorly turgid or pliable. However, turgor must be evaluated in relation to the degree of dehydration. Thus, specific documentation may describe skin turgor as: good or normal, decreased, poor, or doughy. Briskly responsive, pliable skin is diagnosed as normal.

The presence of poor or doughy skin turgor should produce a closer examination for other signs of dehydration. Ideally, the degree of dehydration should be determined. Dehydration is classified as follows: mild= (6% to 8% fluid loss), moderate= (10% to 12% fluid loss), and severe= (12% to 15% fluid loss). Regions of the body that have an excessive amount of skin are not good candidates to test for turgor. Therefore, the cervical area will not produce valuable information.

A complete physical examination should also include the detection of any fleas, lice, mites, ticks, or lesions. The technician should examine the animal by palpation — described as a gentle pressure applied by the fingers over the animal's body. This should be useful in detecting lumps, swellings, and in producing reactions to painful points that the patient may be experiencing. Any unusual masses or changes in organ size, or other tissue enlargements, should be recorded. These observations will be used to further determine the patient's overall health. Indeed, all available information should be used to diagnose and treat the patient fully and properly.

Eyes, ears, and nares
The animal should also be examined for proper reflexes and appropriate responses to visual stimuli. This is essential in determining problems associated with the eyes. Likewise, the technician should record any leakage or matter that is released from the eyes. The color of this leakage may be clear or purulent. Purulent describes an exudate that contains pus or a similar yellowish or greenish fluid. This may indicate an infection in the animal.

The examination should note any irregularities in the cornea. Likewise, the clarity of the conjunctiva (the membrane covering the eye's surface) and the color of the sclera (the whites of the eyes) are both noted. The technician will manipulate the ear in checking its health. The technician will note any auditory stimuli response, abnormal or disproportionate odor, and the presence or absence of matter in the ear canal.

The technician will note the quality of any movements involving the patient's head. Any favoring of one side, disequilibrium, poor coordination, etc, should be recorded. The technician will check the nares or nostrils. The color and consistency of mucus released in the nasal region should be noted. This includes any sneezing or congestion observed. The nostrils should also be checked for any obstructions that may be causing a congested response.

Gastrointestinal system
The technician will appraise the gastrointestinal system by checking the animal's mouth, teeth, and gums. The technician should make a note of all fractured, missing, or discolored teeth found in the animal's mouth. The animal's gums should be inspected for periodontal disease. Likewise, the presence of halitosis (bad breath) should be recorded. The technician will also make notes regarding any signs of malocclusion or unusual alignment of the teeth. The technician will seek to determine the age of the animal as related to dental status and overall health.

The animal's tonsils should be examined for any growth or excess size. In addition, the technician should document any disproportionate salivation or problems associated with swallowing. The technician will record any greenish- or yellowish-colored mucus. The mucous membranes should be pale pink in color to be considered normal. Any irregularities should be recorded. The gingival tissue should be checked for capillary refill time (abbreviated as CRT). This can be examined by applying gentle pressure on the gums and then quickly releasing in order to determine how long the gum tissue takes to return to a normal color. The refill process should be brisk and uniform in its resaturation.

Respiratory system
The technician will need to listen to the patient's internal organs with a stethoscope. This is referred to as auscultation. For pulmonary auscultation the stethoscope should be placed on the back or the side of the thorax. The thorax is located between the neck and the abdomen. Moving the stethoscope to various points throughout the thoracic area can aid in obtaining a complete evaluation of the upper and lower lobes of the lungs and the trachea. This may be particularly important with larger animals. The technician should listen closely for any sounds that are irregular. This can involve crackling, wheezing, stridor, rhonchi, or rales. Stridor refers to a severe, struggling, high-pitched gasping for air, arising from an obstructed or highly constricted airway. Rhonchi are wet, mucus-laden wheezing or snoring sounds. Rales refer to a crackling, bubbling sound that emanates from the chest region. Some sounds may present only at the time of inspiration or expiration, with others present during both inspiration and expiration.

Sounds coming from the animal's upper airway and trachea should be checked further, particularly if an obstruction appears to be involved. Likewise, any problematic breathing should be noted. The animal's respiratory pattern, rate, and depth, and any changes noted with exertion may be important. The animal may exhibit hyperventilation or hypoventilation, panting or shallow breathing, and dyspnea. Hyperventilation refers to a deep, quick-paced breathing that may be induced by anxiety or by an organic disease process. In particular, the disease of an organ may contribute to problems associated with carbon dioxide levels in the blood. The animal may then experience dizziness or weakness.

Hypoventilation refers to a shallow breathing that that allows carbon dioxide to build up in the bloodstream. Dyspnea refers to difficult or labored breathing, often associated with heart disease coupled with overexertion. These problematic symptoms should be recorded. Felines that exhibit quick, shallow breaths or open-mouth breathing may be in physiological distress. This observation should be carefully noted to further promote the proper diagnosis of the animal.

Routes of drug administration

Oral
The patient should be given medication by mouth in an oral dosage that is liquid, semisolid, or in a pill or capsule form. Liquid medication can be injected in the pocket of the cheek via a dropper or syringe. The pill or capsules should be positioned towards the back of the animal's tongue. This is accomplished with one hand, while the other hand works to keep the animal's mouth open. Once the pill has been positioned, then the animal's mouth is held closed until the animal has swallowed noticeably. The animal cannot be given an oral medication if there

are certain adverse conditions present. Contraindicating adverse conditions include vomiting, injury in the oral cavity or esophagus, or problematic swallowing. In these situations the use of oral medication is contraindicated and highly inadvisable.

Topical

Other medications may be applied topically. These medications can be placed on or rubbed into the skin. The animal's skin must be sanitized and clipped of any hair in any region to be used for medication application. This must be done before any medication is applied to the area. However, it is perfectly acceptable to place appropriate topical medications directly on any lesions or wounds. The directions accompanying each medication will provide specific information regarding the amounts recommended to be applied at any given time. In addition, the directions should note the time it takes for the medication to be absorbed. The technician that applies the medication should wear gloves to prevent accidental absorption into the skin.

Parenteral

Some drugs are best delivered through an injection. All drugs taken by any means other than via the digestive system (i.e., by way of skin absorption, inhalation, injections, etc) are referred to as parenteral medications. However, the term is most often used in reference to injectable drugs (whether administered by syringe, IV, or other infusion method). Medications by injection typically take effect much more quickly, will not be regurgitated or expectorated, and are more completely absorbed into the system than drugs administered orally.

There are 3 ways that an injectable drug can be administered by parenteral means. These 3 routes are subcutaneous, intramuscular, and intravenous. Subcutaneous is abbreviated as SC or SQ. Intramuscular is abbreviated as IM. Intravenous is abbreviated as IV. However, there are additional distinctions which may be involved, including intradermal, intraperitoneal, intracardiac, intratracheal, intramedullary or intraosseous, intranasal, intrathecal, and intra-arterial. Intradermal (between skin layers) is abbreviated as ID. Intraperitoneal (into the abdominal cavity) is abbreviated as IP. Intracardiac (into the heart) is abbreviated as IC. Intratracheal (into the trachea) is abbreviated as IT. Intramedullary or intraosseous (into a bone) is abbreviated as IO. Intranasal (into the nose) is abbreviated as IN. Intrathecal (into the space around the spinal cord) is also abbreviated as IT, and thus is context specific. Intra-arterial (into an artery) is abbreviated as IA.

In most cases, SC injections are given with a 22 to 25 gauge needle. SC injections are often administered in the back of the hips or neck of an animal. This is an ideal location due to the excess skin found in these regions. Vaccinations are normally given in subcutaneous injections under the skin.

IM injections are given with a 22 to 25 gauge needle. The injection is administered into the lumbar muscles or bicep femoris muscle. This injection is delivered in a volume that is no more than about 2 mL in any one location. Therefore, a number of sites may be needed to obtain the desired effect. IV administrations can be given in the cephalic, femoral, saphenous, or jugular veins. The IV is the quickest route to produce the desired effect. This also is an ideal method when a large dose of medication or fluid must be given. The cephalic region refers to the area within or on the head. The femoral region refers to the area of the thigh or the femur. The saphenous vein is found in the leg and refers to 2 major veins which travel from the foot to the thigh. The jugular vein refers to one of the 4 main pairs of veins found in the neck

Fluid balance and abnormal fluid loss

The body is uniquely designed to maintain a proper balance of fluids and other biochemistries. This design incorporates a body makeup of about 60% water. The amount of water is divided between intracellular and extracellular components within the body. However, this constant need to maintain a fluid balance must be met by metabolic functions and by the restoration of lost fluid through oral means. The act of drinking restores fluid by oral means. Then, the body's metabolism plays a part in how that fluid is allocated, maintained, and utilized. Some metabolic functions include losing fluids through respiration, excretion, and episodic routines such as sweating and milk production.

Furthermore, fluid can be lost by atypical adverse conditions. These adverse conditions may include the following: vomiting, diarrhea, and/or abnormally excessive urination. Some diseases induce polyuria (excessive urination). Available fluids may also be reduced due to the patient's state of health. For example, chronic disease or severe injury can negatively impact the patient's ability to take in fluids. Ill dogs that have rapid respiration or excessive panting may also suffer from further fluid loss.

Dehydration

The animal must also be carefully checked to determine the degree of dehydration. The following factors should be considered in that determination: weight (especially recent rapid changes likely due to fluid loss), skin turgor, moistness of mucous membranes, heart rate, and CRT (capillary refill time). These factors must be evaluated through a physical inspection of the animal. Animals with a rate of dehydration under 5% of total normal fluid status do not typically show obvious signs or symptoms. However, animals with rates of 5% to 6% dehydration will usually exhibit a mild degree of skin turgor evidenced by a lack of pliability to the skin. Animals with 8% dehydration will exhibit a more moderate rate of skin turgor, a minor rise in CRT, and some dryness in the mucous membranes. The CRT can be examined by applying gentle pressure on the gums and then quickly releasing in order to determine how long the gum tissue takes to return to a normal color. The refill process should normally be brisk and uniform in its resaturation of the gum tissue.

Animals with dehydration rates of 10% to 12% total body fluid loss will exhibit moderate to severe skin turgor, hollow-looking eyes, a marked rise in CRT (capillary refill time), dry mucous membranes, rapid heart and respiratory rates, cold limbs, and perhaps signs of shock. The CRT can be examined by applying gentle pressure on the gums and then quickly releasing in order to determine how long the gum tissue takes to return to a normal color. The refill process should normally be brisk and uniform in its resaturation of the gum tissue. The animal exhibiting 12% to 15% dehydration will be extremely metabolically depressed. In addition, the animal will likely already be in shock. This animal is in danger of dying from the severe level of dehydration and shock. Tests can be given to come to a determination about the degree of dehydration present. A dehydration test measures the packed cell volume or PCV, total plasma protein or TPP levels, urine-specific gravity, and a lower rate of urine production. The degree of dehydration should be classified as follows: mild (6% to 8%), moderate (10% to 12%), and severe (12% to 15%).

Fluid replacement

Fluid levels must be promptly replaced in patients that are suffering from hypovolemic shock, or severely dehydrated conditions. These patients should receive 60 to 90 mL/kg/hr of fluids to replace the lost volume. The replacement fluids should be given to the patient over a 12- to 24-hour time frame in order to avoid inducing other problems. The total fluid amount needing to be replaced can be calculated by determining the daily fluid requirements. The calculation for the amount of replacement fluids required is the percent dehydration (as a decimal point figure) multiplied by the animal's body weight in kg, multiplied by 1000 to obtain the replacement amount in milliliters.

The quantity of maintenance fluid needed is approximately 40 to 60 mL/kg/day. A measurement must be taken to determine the volume of urine excreted on a daily basis. In addition, diarrhea, vomitus, and other concurrently lost fluids should be measured. This includes any fluid that drains from an injury. This provides an estimated amount of the total fluid needed to provide rehydration, maintenance, and replacement fluid for that which is continuously excreted in one form or another. Replacement solutions include Normosol R and lactated Ringer's solution or LRS. Maintenance solutions are known as: Normosol M and normal saline with KCl.

Contraindications
There are times when an animal's immediate condition may make it inadvisable to pursue rapid fluid replacement. For example, pulmonary edema may make rehydration problematic. Pulmonary edema is an excess of fluid accumulating in the lungs. This is a concern that requires regular and frequent observations until all troubling fluid dynamics can be adequately addressed and resolved. Other problems that may make rapid fluid replacement therapy inadvisable include: pulmonary contusions, brain injury, severe ascites, cerebral edema from any cause, and congestive heart failure. If the animal shows signs of over-hydration, then fluid therapy must be halted. Over-hydration symptoms include: restlessness, an elevated respiratory rate, wheezing or other sounds of respiratory compromise emanating from the lungs, an abnormal rise in blood pressure, chemosis, and pitting edema. Chemosis is demonstrated by an enlargement or swelling of the eye whites. Pitting edema is a sign of fluid overload in the extremities, seen when the tissues are firmly pressed and do not rebound (leaving a "pit" or dent where previously pressed). At the conclusion of fluid replacement therapy the animal is again evaluated. The weight of the animal should be taken. The specific gravity and amount of any recent urine voiding should also be noted. The recorded amounts,

patient reactions, and veterinarian's instructions are applied in making any changes needed for further fluid therapy.

Routes of fluid administration

Fluids can be given to a patient in a number of ways. Fluids can be given through oral, subcutaneous, percutaneous, intravenous, or intramedullary routes into the body. A syringe or a feeding tube is often used in the administration of fluids by oral means. However, an oral administration route is not advisable in animals displaying certain adverse conditions. These include: vomiting, esophageal injury, and/or pancreatitis. Pancreatitis exists when the digestive and endocrine gland known as the pancreas becomes inflamed and swollen.

A subcutaneous fluid replacement route is often used in cases that exhibit symptoms of mild dehydration. However, the subcutaneous fluid route cannot be applied if the patient is in shock or in cases of severe dehydration. This is due to the relatively slow rate of absorption associated with poor peripheral circulation, which is a symptom of shock. Therefore, it is best to administer intravenous fluids to patients in shock accompanied by moderate to severe dehydration. Younger animals, or those that are very small, should be given fluids by intramedullary infusion. This method allows the fluid to be absorbed quickly, since it is delivered directly into the highly vascularized bone marrow.

Canine blood donor requirements

Dogs are classified into 2 blood types: Type A- (A negative) or Type A+ (A positive). The A- blood type is regarded as the universal blood donor type for dogs. This is because all dogs, whether they are A- or A+, can tolerate receiving this blood type via transfusion, while A+ blood is only well tolerated by dogs that are also A+ in blood type. A blood donor gives blood to another patient in need. The ideal donor can be found among any breed of dog. Further, the ideal donor can be either male or female. However, the animal should have been neutered or spayed, to reduce blood hormone levels. Neutering is defined as the surgical removal of the animal's testicles or ovaries. In addition, the animal's weight is a factor. It should be larger than 25 kg or 55 lb. Age is also a factor. It should be between the age of 1 and 7 years old. The animal should have received all of its vaccinations. The donor's blood type should already have been determined. The animal should have the following additional tests on a yearly basis: blood chemistry, CBC, and urinalysis. The ideal donor should receive a normal result from these 3 tests before the blood is extracted.

A blood donor animal requires regular checkups and tests to allow the doctor the opportunity to gauge whether or not the donor animal remains a suitable candidate. These checkups should be scheduled at 6-month intervals. The checkups should be used to detect parasites in the animal, among other health conditions. Of particular importance is an evaluation regarding the presence of heartworms or intestinal parasites. The presence of any infectious diseases will rule out the donor's suitability for giving blood. Infectious diseases include the blood parasites, and other parasites responsible for rickettsial diseases. The primary blood parasites are Babesia canis and Hemobartonella canis. The parasites responsible for rickettsial diseases include Ehrlichia canis, Ehrlichia platus, Borrelia burgdorferi and Rickettsia rickettsii. The rickettsial parasites are primarily transmitted through ticks. Ticks are defined as blood-sucking insects that burrow into the skin. These insects have the ability to attach themselves to humans and animals. Therefore, it is important to check the animal's skin thoroughly for any signs of ticks after being outdoors. The canine blood donor should fast before giving blood to reduce the likelihood of producing a lipemic (fat or lipid laden) blood specimen.

Canine blood collection procedures

The procedure for preparing a blood donor begins with a sedative. The animal is given a sedative suitable for the canine species. The animal is then placed in a lateral recumbent position with its neck stretched out for the procedure. This position allows easy access to the jugular vein. The jugular vein is ideal for withdrawing the blood from the patient. The cephalic vein is also concurrently used to give the animal needed replacement fluids. Both the cephalic vein and the jugular vein are in need of preparation before commencing the blood withdrawal. The preparation includes clipping the hair in the area of venipuncture. A catheter is a thin tube that is used to inject fluid into the cephalic vein. The blood is drawn out of the jugular vein by means of a 16 gauge needle. The blood is collected in a bag that holds an anticoagulant. A full collection of blood is measured at 450 mL.

A scale is applied to gain an exact measurement of the blood collected. This exact measurement is used to ensure that the collection bag is not filled too much or too little. A full collection of blood is measured at 450 mL. There is a risk to the animal of developing a hematoma (a clotted mass of blood) at the jugular venipuncture site. This risk can be diminished by placing a firm, but gentle force directly on the jugular vein for 2 minutes following the closing stages of blood withdrawal. In addition, it is advisable to only take a maximum of 10 to 20 mL/kg at an interval of at least 3 weeks. The veterinarian should make every effort to replace the blood extracted with fluids given at rates measuring 3x the volume of blood lost. The replacement fluids should be administered to the patient via a catheter through the cephalic vein in the region of the patient's head.

Feline blood donor requirements

There are 3 kinds of feline blood types. The 3 types are known as Type A, Type B, and Type AB. Type A is the most common type found in domesticated cats. This is true of both longhair and shorthair species. However, purebreds most often have the blood type known as Type B. It is not necessary to determine the type of blood in the feline before the blood withdrawal procedure. The ideal feline blood donor will be under 8 years of age. The cat will be neutered or spayed. The cat will have received all of its vaccinations. In addition, the cat will not be overweight or underweight. The ideal weight for the cat is a lean body mass of not lower than 4.5 kg or 10 lb. The cat with a good disposition and that has been accustomed to living indoors will usually find the procedure to be less traumatic.

Feline blood collection procedures

The first step in preparing the cat is to clip the hair away from the jugular and the cephalic vein regions. The next step involves providing an aseptic cleansing to the regions involved. The animal should next be given a sedative. The cat is then placed in a lateral recumbent or sternal recumbent position. A 19 gauge butterfly needle is inserted into the jugular vein. To diminish the movement associated with the needle in the jugular vein, the staff should utilize a 60 mL syringe with 8.5 mL of anticoagulant joined with a flexible phlebotomy tube to the butterfly needle. In addition, the staff should maintain a focus on the animal's vital signs, including its pulse, respiration, and blood pressure throughout the procedure. Partway through, the cat should be given replacement fluids. The blood and anticoagulant should be mixed often. The withdrawal should be finalized at the time that the 60 mL syringe is measured in its fullness. This is followed by the removal of the butterfly needle. Then, the staff places pressure on the jugular vein to prevent a hematoma or blood clot from developing. The replacement fluid is completed at 180 mL, or 3 times the amount of blood extracted.

Fresh whole blood, packed red blood cells, and plasma

Fresh whole blood is given when an animal exhibits one or more of the following: hemorrhagic shock, anemia, excessive surgical hemorrhage, clotting disorders, non-immune-mediated hemolytic anemia, and sometimes immune-mediated hemolytic anemia. Crystalloid (an isotonic or hypertonic fluid, such as Lactated Ringer's solution, used as a blood volume expander) is given in combination with packed red blood cells (RBCs) when it becomes necessary to maintain the animal's fluid balance and osmotic pressure. Packed RBCs can be given to the animal that has suffered from hemolytic and nonregenerative anemias. RBCs may be maintained in an "extender" solution such as ADSOL (adenine, glucose, mannitol, and sodium chloride). Packed RBCs stored in ADSOL will naturally have a greater total volume than packed RBCs stored alone. Further, the unit volume of RBCs packed in other preservatives (i.e., Optisol or Nutricel, etc) may vary from that of ADSOL. However, the cell count per unit should be the same regardless of the solution used. When mixing packed RBCs with ADSOL, add the solution to the cells rather than the cells to the solution. This reduces the degree of hemolysis during and after mixing. The shock and burn patient can benefit from a plasma transfusion. This type of transfusion will supply volume replacement when tissue-based fluids are lost in the absence of skin. In addition, other medical conditions such as hypoproteinemia, pancreatitis, and sepsis can benefit from this type of transfusion.

Electrical impulses of the heart

The heart organ is motivated by an electrical impulse which works to cause the tightening and the relaxing of the heart muscle. This tightening or contraction is referred to as cardiac systole, or the systolic phase. The relaxation or loosening of the muscle is known as diastole, or the diastolic phase. These phases describe the heartbeat or continuous pulsation of the heart muscle that is responsible for the circulation of blood throughout the body. The contraction of the myocardium (systole) is immediately preceded by (and thus is sometimes referred to as) depolarization. In like manner, the relaxation of the myocardium may be referred to as repolarization. The electrical impulse is transmitted through the regions of the heart in a systematic, recurring pattern. Electrical activity begins at the point known as the sinoatrial node. Another term for the sinoatrial node is the cardiac pacemaker. It consists of a small mass of fibers positioned in the heart's right atrium. The heart's cells are all closely linked. This linkage allows the depolarization and repolarization to move along at a rapid pace.

The electrical activity is carried by various nerve fiber bundles from the sinoatrial node to the right and left atria and then toward the ventricles. The electrical activity continues until it reaches the atrioventricular (AV) node. The AV node is the junction where the atria and the ventricles are interconnected. The AV node produces a brief transmission delay once activated. This allows the ventricles a momentary period of time to fill with blood prior to a contraction. The ventricles are the lower, larger chambers of the heart. The atria are the upper, smaller chambers of the heart that serve solely to fill the ventricles in preparation for significant blood movement through the lungs or body. Depolarization spreads through the interventricular system between heartbeats. It moves through the left and right bundle branches. At the apex or tip of the heart, the Purkinje Fibers or neuroelectrical conduction branches finally end. The impulse transmission then radiates upward and outward through the ventricles, producing a smooth, upward rippling, milking-like contraction. Effective cardiac contraction is vital, as it causes the blood to be pumped into the arteries on its way to the lungs or throughout the entire body.

Electrocardiography

Non-invasive electrocardiography can be accomplished through the use of bioelectrical leads placed in such a way as to externally sense the heart's electrical conduction activity. The device is used in making a profile of the electrical impulses that govern and regulate the function of the heart. Each impulse is given immediately prior to various areas of the heart experiencing muscle contraction or movement.

The electrocardiograph gathers signals through the use of a voltmeter that has the capacity to gauge the amount of electricity that radiates through electrodes positioned on the outside of the person's chest. The signal is recorded ("traced") on a continuous roll of thermograph paper, which provides a permanent record of the electrocardiogram. The abbreviation for electrocardiogram is ECG (or EKG, to differentiate it from the ultrasonographic abbreviation for an echocardiogram). ECG tracings are visible when drawn by a heated stylus on heat-sensitive graph paper, or as transiently displayed on a monitor screen. The ECG is capable of measuring the amplitude or strength of electrical activity, and the duration or length of time associated with each electrical impulse. Normal heart contractions are recorded and viewed as normal rhythms on the ECG.

<u>ECG waveform</u>
The electrocardiogram may be described as a graph-based display and recording of the heart's electrical functions. This graphic display is produced by way of an electrocardiograph instrument. The electrical activity induces motion in a tracing stylus that then produces a line drawing of a continuous wave tracing of electrical activity. The continuous line drawing of

linked sequences of electrical impulses transmitted across the heart constitutes the electrocardiogram or ECG.

The series of electrical events that begin and end a single heartbeat is referred to as waves, complexes, and intervals. For purposes of evaluation, the electrical activities of a heartbeat are broken into 4 parts. These 4 parts are known as the P wave, the PR interval, the QRS complex, and the T wave. The P wave is a result of the depolarization that takes place in the right and left atrium. The P wave lasts for about 0.12 seconds or less. The section of the ECG that begins with the atrial depolarization (the P wave), to the point known as the ventricular depolarization (the QRS complex), is referred to as the PR interval. The PR interval is described as a breadth of time that can range from 0.12 to 0.20 seconds. The QRS complex is a result of the ventricular depolarization (contraction). The QRS complex typically lasts between 0.04 to 0.12 seconds. Repolarization of the ventricular myocardium can be viewed in a segment of the graph-based tracing of the ECG. This segment is known as the T wave. Atrial repolarization activity is overshadowed by the QRS complex. Thus, it cannot be viewed on the tracings represented in an ECG.

Supplies and procedures
When performing an ECG the patient should be given a protective coverlet, and cushion or mat to reduce the harmful effects associated with a steel table's ability to conduct electricity. The patient should be swabbed with alcohol, conducting gel, or paste. These substances give a boost to skin where contact is made. Some machines designed for taking human ECGs can be adapted for use with animals. Necessary modifications include the use of a filed or bent alligator clip. This modification inhibits the pinching or bruising that is often associated with the use of strong alligator clips applied directly to the skin. In addition, the continuous monitoring offered by pads (applied to shaved skin) or even subcutaneous wires can also be employed.

Electrical signals from the heart can be conveyed to the electrocardiograph in many ways, including: 1) by wireless ECG devices positioned near the animal; 2) by use of adhesive ECG pads; 3) by rubber straps holding small metal plates to the skin; or 4) by the subcutaneous placement of ECG wires. Each method has advantages and disadvantages. If pads are used, the pad is placed directly on the animal's bare skin. The animal's fur is clipped to allow complete contact. If alligator skin clips are used, they may be clipped directly to the animal's skin. However, this technique can be painful. Other techniques may provide the animal with a less traumatic experience. Where necessary, (particularly for long-term monitoring) ECG wires can be placed subcutaneously. The placement of surgical wire can be accomplished after cleaning the area. The wire is cleansed with alcohol. Then, a 20 gauge needle is used to introduce the wire under the skin. The ends of the wire are bent along one end and adhesive tape is applied. This is done to prevent harm in long-haired animals. In addition, this method allows easy removal of the wire following the procedure.
During the ECG recording process the animal can be placed into a right lateral recumbent position. Some larger sized animals may remain in an upright position on their feet. Cats are normally more comfortable in a crouch position on the table. Regardless, the animal requires manual restraints.

Keeping each limb from touching the other body parts will reduce the contact of skin upon skin. This is important for an accurate ECG reading. Leads are fastened at the center point or proximal left and right of the elbow bone or olecranon processes. Leads can also be fastened to the center point or proximal left and right stifles of the hind leg and the chest. This includes the dorsal or the back of the thorax near the seventh thoracic vertebra in the chest region. A sedative should help an animal that is overly anxious or unruly.

It is usually best to take a standard recording with the paper speed set at 25 mm/sec. Typically, 30 cm or 12 inches for each lead is recorded for an ECG that incorporates all the necessary information for proper evaluation. The paper speed is often set at 50 cm/sec for small dogs and cats. Various animals with faster or slower heart rates may require different paper speeds to provide adequate tracing differentiation and clarity. The ECG tracing should also incorporate pertinent patient identification and procedural information including: the date of the ECG, patient name and species, client name, and any other relevant information.

Interpretation
The wave segments denoted as P, Q, R, S, and T are considered the key features of a normal heartbeat. Each QRS complex is associated with a P wave. The P wave has a positive deflection in lead II. However, either a positive or a negative deflection can be associated with the T segment. The PR interval is relatively normal. In most domestic animals, a normal cardiac rhythm can also be referred to as a sinus rhythm. The measured values should be examined for similarities and differences in association with the normal values as denoted by each species of animal. This comparison should take place at the end of a complete ECG. The complexes should be evaluated by the veterinarian or a trained technician. The number of complexes in a 3 second period should be counted. This will allow the professional to also determine the heart rate of the animal examined.

Sinus arrhythmia

Sinus arrhythmia (also called respiratory sinus arrhythmia or RSA) refers to a normal variation in heartbeat, as influenced by respiratory patterns. Both inspiratory and expiratory respirations can alter the heart's sinus rhythm. Typically, the heart rate increases during inspiration and decreases during expiration. Theorists suggest that this maximizes cardiac output during more effective ventilatory periods. Variations are more pronounced in younger animals and moderate with age. The "sinus" term refers to the sinus node (or the sinoatrial node), which is the heart's natural pacemaker. It is important to know of respiratory sinus arrhythmia, as these changes will be apparent during an ECG. Neurologically induced cardiac variations (as seen in altered vagal tone and parasympathetic system responses, including emotions) can also contribute to the magnitude of sinus arrhythmia experienced. Finally, any respiratory disease in an animal may also bring about an altered sinus arrhythmia.

Sinus bradycardia

A particularly slow but regular ventricular heart rate can be described as sinus bradycardia. This term is generally used when the heart rate is less than 70 beats per minute for dogs that weigh under 20 kg or 45 lb. This rate is also given for dogs that have a heart rate less than 60 beats per minute when weighing over 20 kg or 45 lb. Heart rates measured at 100 beats per minute or less are indicative of sinus bradycardia in cats. Animals experiencing profound bradycardia can exhibit symptoms such as weakness, hypotension, and syncope. Both excessive and reduced parasympathetic tone may result in sinus bradycardia. Sinus bradycardia can sometimes also be attributed to respiratory disease. The disease can cause the animal to experience a number of problems, including struggling to draw in air, gastric irritation, increased cerebrospinal fluid pressure, hypothyroidism, hypothermia, hyperkalemia, and hypoglycemia. Certain drug therapies may also induce the condition.

Orogastric intubation

Orogastric intubation is described as a method employed to purge the stomach of its contents. This method can also be employed to dispense food or nutrients to animals that have been orphaned at a young age. In particular this may include neonate animals, usually less than one month of age. In addition, orogastric intubation can be employed to flush out stomach contents with a flow of water in a gastric lavage. Finally, it can also be used to distribute medications or radiographic contrast agents, such as barium, into the abdominal and gastrointestinal regions.

The veterinarian will need to use a variety of supplies when performing an orogastric intubation. The supplies include a stomach tube, speculum, adhesive tape, and a lubricant. Smaller animals such as puppies and kittens will require a 12 F to 18 F infant feeding tube. Larger dogs, ranging over 10 kg or 22.2 lb, will require an 18 F foal stomach tube.

When performing an orogastric intubation, larger dogs will require a foal stomach tube. To facilitate the intubation process, the medical instrument known as a speculum can be employed. The veterinarian can use a canine speculum to hold the mouth open, or a roll of adhesive tape measuring 1-2 inches wide can be placed crosswise in the mouth to serve as an open speculum when the tube is inserted. The following is also required: an appropriately sized orogastric tube, sterile saline solution in a syringe, tape or a permanent marker for depth marking on the tube, and an appropriate sedative (if needed). If the animal requires any other drugs or substances, these are given via a syringe or a funnel.

Usually, an orogastric intubation does not require sedation. However, in some cases a light tranquilizer can be employed. The animal can remain standing or be positioned in a sternal recumbent position. The tube should be measured against the length of the animal (typically from the mouth to the ninth intercostal space). This will give an approximate length needed to gain access into the stomach of the animal. The oral tip of the tube (i.e., that which will remain immediately outside the mouth) should be designated with tape. Then, the speculum should be introduced into the animal's mouth.

The animal's jaws should be held tightly shut against the speculum by the staff member assigned to the job of restraining the animal. The lubricated tube should be inserted into the mouth opening through the speculum and down to the pre-marked location on the tube. Proper placement should be verified before any fluids or other materials are inserted (typically by withdrawing stomach contents using gentle suction, or by putting 1 mL of sterile water into the tube to cause coughing if pulmonary intubation has occurred). If the tube is found to be located in the trachea, then the tube must be promptly taken out to avoid respiratory compromise and introducing fluids into the lungs. The procedure will have to be repeated until the location is verified as accurate. Once an accurate location has been reached, then necessary fluids and substances can be inserted into the tube. This is followed by a flushing with water, using approximately 6 mL. The tube should not produce any seepage. If this occurs, the seepage can be stopped by placing a thumb over the tube. If this still does not work, then it should be kinked or bent over to stop the flow.

Nasogastric intubation

A nasogastric intubation is described as procedure in which a tube is inserted through the external nares, the nasal cavity, pharynx, and the esophagus, into the stomach region. The veterinarian will typically employ this particular procedure in an effort to supply nutrition in a liquid form to the animal. In addition, this method is suitable for supplying water and other liquids to the animal. A nasogastric tube can be left in place over a long period of time, whereas an orogastric tube cannot. Animals that are anorexic may require lengthy nasogastric feedings if they are extremely thin or unhealthy. Thus, placement of a nasogastric tube can be used to provide the animal with proper nutrition. This may be particularly effective for an anxious animal that is a poor candidate for forced feedings. This procedure also allows the veterinarian a method to introduce medication or a contrast medium into the animal's stomach. One contrast medium that may be used is barium, which is applied in radiology in evaluating the gastrointestinal tract for certain lesions, obstructions, and other problems.

The equipment needed for nasogastric intubation includes a nasogastric feeding tube, a topical ophthalmic anesthetic, lubricating jelly, a syringe, sterile saline solution, injection cap, and any medications or substances needing to be introduced into the patient's stomach. The tube that is employed in the procedure can be of various sizes and materials. For instance, an infant feeding tube can be made from either red rubber or polyurethane. However, the critical elements of this tube are its small diameter and its composition from a flexible material that is soft. Animals that are under 5 kg or 12 pounds require a size 5 F feeding tube. Animals that range in size from 5 to 12 kg or 12-33 pounds require a size 8 F feeding tube. The insertion of the nasogastric intubation also requires a topical ophthalmic anesthetic (to reduce nasal insertion discomfort), lubricating jelly, a syringe containing sterile saline (1 mL), an injection cap, and any medication or liquid to be introduced into the animal's stomach. In some cases, the need for the tube to remain in place for an extended time necessitates that securing dressings be used.

Nasogastric intubation should only be administered to alert patients. Sedation is usually not necessary. The tube is measured first. The tube's measurement consists of the length estimated by assessing the distance between the ninth to thirteenth rib and the nares or nostrils. A topical anesthesia is given at 4 to 5 drops in one nostril. This is followed by the addition of more drops in the same nostril once a period of 2-3 minutes has elapsed. The lubrication of the nasogastric tube is completed at this juncture. The animal's head is then held in one hand. The other hand should be applied to introduce the tube into the anesthetized nostril. The animal must be checked to find out if the tube is properly positioned (stomach versus lungs). This is accomplished by inserting 1 mL of sterile saline into the tube. The animal will cough if the insertion is incorrect. Optionally, gentle suction may be applied until frank stomach contents are aspirated and visualized. Prompt extubation and reinsertion of the tube is necessary if pulmonary intubation has occurred.

The onset of coughing in the animal will be a decisive factor in determining that the tube has been placed in the wrong location. The location is tested by inserting 1mL of sterile saline into the tube. The animal will cough if the tube is in the trachea. This requires that the tube be removed and reinserted. For long-standing tube utilization, the tube should be fastened along the side of the patient's neck with a binding. The tube requires a cap. The cap is essential in keeping the animal from aspirating air into the stomach. Each feeding necessitates that the location of the tube be rechecked. In addition, the tube should be aspirated or suctioned at that time. A finger can be placed over the top of the tube when the tube must be extracted. This keeps any seepage from occurring in the pharynx or throat while the tube is being withdrawn.

Canine urinary catheterization

A urine sample that is free from infective organisms and other contaminants can be used for analysis and cultures. The urine discharge collected in a catheterization tube from the patient should be measured. The urine is most sterile when it is extracted directly from the urinary bladder. A catheterization tube can be used to bring relief to the patient experiencing a urethral obstruction. The catheterization tube can also be used for dispensing medication or contrast media. Contrast media are used in radiology examinations.

A pneumocystography is an example of a test that necessitates a urinary catheterization. The veterinarian should carry out a urinary catheterization on the patient personally. The supplies needed for this procedure include a gentle soap, a sterile urethral catheter, sterile lubricant, and sterile syringes or other sterile collection containers. In addition, female patients require the following: a vaginal speculum, sterile gloves, viscous Xylocaine or 0.5% lidocaine jelly, and possibly a steel catheter. Normally, the catheter is made from polyethylene, vinyl, or rubber. Less flexible and larger catheters can result in a traumatic experience for the patient. Catheters are available in sizes 3.5 F, 5 F, 8 F, and 10 F.

Cystocentesis

Cystocentesis is a needle aspiration technique used to collect a urine sample from a patient. This technique can be applied to cats or dogs. The animal may be in a state of sleepiness or under sedation. The animal should be placed in a dorsal or lateral recumbent position. The bladder should be examined medically and palpated using gentle pressure to detect the fullness of the bladder. Alcohol is wiped over the site where the needle is to be inserted. The veterinarian should prevent any shifting of the bladder with one hand. The other hand is needed to insert the sterile needle and syringe in a caudodorsal direction into the bladder site. It is important to prevent any squeezing pressure from being applied to the bladder during this procedure so as to prevent urine leakage into the peritoneal cavity. The urine is extracted through the syringe with a negative pressure applied on the plunger device. The needle and syringe should then be pulled out of the body as soon as the plunger is released. It is recommended that the sample be immediately transferred to a sanitized, marked container.

Manual compression of the urinary bladder

Manual compression of the urinary bladder can also be used to expel the contents for collection purposes. However, this procedure must not be used if a urinary obstruction is suspected. The urine is collected for inspection of solute concentration, physical properties, and chemical constituents. This unsterile urine sample should not be used for urine cultures. The bladder on the animal can be found by palpating or applying a gentle pressure along the abdomen. This pressure should begin at the site where the very last rib is located. The examination should be carried out by moving from the front to the rear portion of the body in a caudal direction. Another technique used in locating the bladder consists of palpating along the upper portion of the rear legs. The movement starts at the back of the body and continues along towards the front lower portion of the body. Once located, pressure should be applied lightly over the bladder in a sustained or continuous manner to allow the urine to be expelled from the bladder. The expelled urine is then promptly transferred into a sterile container. Following this the urine sample can be analyzed.

Wound healing

There are 4 phases associated with wound healing: inflammatory, débridement, repair, and maturation. The inflammatory phase is the initial phase that follows an injury. This phase is associated with the appearance of scabs. Scabs are a crust over the injured area. This dried substance can be formed from blood, serum, and pus. This crust protects the wound so that healing can begin. The débridement phase commences about 6 hours after the injury takes place. Neutrophils and monocytes work to remove foreign material, bacteria, and necrotic tissue from the wound. Both neutrophils and monocytes can be described as white blood cells. In most cases, the repair phase starts within approximately 3 to 5 days after the initial wound. However, the time associated with this phase is contingent upon foreign substances being adequately extracted from the infected area. The final phase is known as maturation. Maturation can extend for a number of years (i.e., to include scar lightening, etc). Refashioning the collagen fibers and other fibrous tissue promotes complete wound recovery.

Multiple phases may sometimes operate simultaneously, accomplished by a series of overlapping actions.

Wound treatment

Appropriate wound treatment involves protective measures, evaluation, and treatment. The initial protective measure requires that the wound be covered with a dressing and/or a splint of some sort. The second step involves an evaluation of the wound's degree of severity. The most severe cases are those that require control of hemorrhaging. Once any hemorrhaging is under control, the wound should be checked to lessen further contamination and infection risks. Hair or other debris should be cleaned and clipped away from the area. The border surrounding the wound should be thoroughly cleansed with an antimicrobial/detergent scrub. This step also involves washing out any hollow body parts or organs. Getting rid of necrotic tissue is the step known as débridement. This is necessary so that new tissue can grow over the wound. Necrotic tissue would hinder this process. In addition, it may be necessary to place a drainage tube to allow excess air and fluid to exit the wound site.

Bandages

Types of absorptions
There are 3 types of bandages used on a wound. These include: dry-to-dry bandages, wet-to-dry bandages, and wet-to-wet bandages. Loose necrotic tissue should be addressed with a dry-to-dry bandage. The dry gauze stays in place with the follow-up application of a dry, absorbent wrap. The patient will experience pain whenever the bandage is removed, but dead and dying tissue is naturally débrided and removed with it.

It is best to use a wet-to-dry bandage on any infected or open wounds. If an exuded substance is present then the wound may require a wet, saline-moistened or medicated bandage placed inside and dry bandage coverings outside. This type of bandage is advantageous as it is able to treat infection and still absorb exudates that emanate from the wound. This type of bandage can also reduce pain associated with the removal of exuded substances attached to the binding. The bandages soak up excess fluid from the wound. The bindings are not taken off of the patient when wet. Wet-to-wet dressings can sometimes be useful for chronic wounds or for larger, ulcerated wounds that require internal tissue regrowth before epidermal tissue can grow and provide protective coverage. Deep pressure sores are one possible example. This form of bandage is removed while still wet.

Layers
The 3 principal layers of bandages are the non-adhesive primary layer, the secondary layer, and the tertiary layer. The non-adhesive primary layer is used without anything in between it and the wound. The type of tissue that forms over a wound, known as granulated tissue, should be treated with a non-adhesive primary layer. This bandage layer prevents further trauma to the injury site. Exuded substances are soaked up by the cushioned, secondary layer. Common name brands include Kling or Sof-Kling. Finally, the exterior layer is known as the tertiary layer. This layer gives the 2 bottom layers more reinforcement. This

- 19 -

reinforcement is due to the type of bandage used, including adhesive tapes, elastic bandages, Vet Wrap (3M), and conforming stretch gauze. The adhesive tape gives the bandage the ability to bond to the other layers. The elastic bandage and stretch gauze is expandable and flexible over the layers covering the wound.

Reasons and precautions for bandaging

Head and neck

The patient's head and neck may require a protective bandage after certain surgeries. The following surgeries are associated with this need: postocular surgery, aural hematoma repair, and ear surgery. In addition, a bandage of this type may be needed to firmly secure a jugular catheter or a nasogastric or pharyngostomy tube into place. Wound edema is a condition in which serous fluid builds up in excessive amounts in the patient. In the head and neck area, this condition can endanger the patient's life. Therefore, the condition of the wound and surrounding swelling should be checked often. This may require removal of the bandage to allow an inspection of the site. The patient's respiration, skin color, and involved mucous membranes should be carefully checked. The bandage should be slack enough to allow the insertion of 2 fingers underneath the bindings. Patients with respiratory concerns should have their bindings loosened. It may be necessary to reapply a different bandage. Animals that are opposed to wearing a head or neck bandage may need to be given an Elizabethan collar. The Elizabethan collar is used to prevent the animal's access to the bandaging material.

Limbs

A patient's limbs may require bandaging for a variety of reasons. These reasons include: to reduce or stop movement (i.e., in bone fractures), to keep a wound safe from infection or further contaminants, and to maintain the positioning and stability of a limb for purposes of fluid therapy (i.e., a subcutaneous infusion or IV line, etc).

The best bandage application provides an even distribution of pressure throughout the bandaged area of the limb. Equitably distributed pressure ensures reasonably unimpeded circulation in the limb. In addition, the entire limb requires a bandage whenever the upper sector of the appendage has been injured. Otherwise, continued movement in the lower area of the appendage may impair healing in the upper area. Whenever an extremity bandage has been placed, it is necessary to carefully ensure adequate circulation. Symptoms of impaired circulation include: swelling around the toes, coldness to touch, and paleness around the nail beds. This requires prompt readjustment and loosening of the bandage. Ideally, when sufficiently loose, 2 fingers can be inserted beneath the binding. The animal's bandage should be covered with a protective bag such as an ordinary plastic bag, a rubber glove, or unfilled fluid bag whenever the animal is up and about. This covering should help keep the binding unsoiled and dry. This covering can be secured for a short time by affixing one end of the protective bag to the proximal end of the appendage.

Tail

There may be occasions when an animal's tail may also require a bandage. This bandage should incorporate and be able to cover the animal's wound. An animal that has had a tumor removed or a partial tail amputation will also benefit from the application of a bandage. An animal experiencing a period of persistent diarrhea may also benefit from the application of a tail bandage. This bandage can bundle up both the appendage and any associated hair, and thereby better help in securing and maintaining the cleanliness of the animal at this difficult time. An amputation can involve persistent bleeding. This bleeding can be induced, exacerbated, and/or perpetuated by excessive tail wagging or by bringing the intact portion of the tail in contact with a hard object. Tail wagging movements can be reduced by sedating the animal. However, this is only a temporizing intervention and one of last resort, due to the negative effects of such medication. An optional way to lessen tail movement is to slide a tube-shaped item over the bottom of the remaining portion of the tail. This should reduce the momentum of the tail wagging, and provide some additional protection to the animal's tail. Analgesics or painkillers can also be given to the patient to reduce the animal's distress and painful symptoms.

Tumors

Benign and malignant

A growth may be described as either benign (non-cancerous) or malignant (cancerous). Cancer is often defined in terms of the tumor site, the severity, and the type of tissue in which the growth is located. Other terms often used to describe a growth include mass, lump, lesion, neoplasm, tumor, and malignancy. The least severe cancerous tumor is one that is described as "localized". Localized tumors have not spread to other parts of the body. These tumors are often fairly simple to remove if they are also encapsulated (i.e., a lump with clear margins), but may be more difficult if they are diffuse (fuzzy, or tentacle-like). Normally, the primary danger associated with a benign tumor is derived from the place it occupies inside the body. A tumor can obstruct or prevent the body from performing normally, and thus can be dangerous or even life-threatening. More serious tumors are those described as both cancerous and metastatic. These types of tumors are invasive and malignant. These cancer cells often break free and move into a secondary region of the body. The regions frequently involved include the lymph nodes, bones, lungs, and other internal organs. This spreading of cells from the primary site to the secondary position is known as metastasis. These locations need not have any relative connection. The terms primary and secondary are used only to designate the original tumor as opposed to any that later emerge if the cancer spreads.

Classification

Tumors can be described as either benign or malignant and are often classified according to origination site, severity, and tissue type involved. Sarcomas are classified as a malignancy that grows in muscle, tendon, bone, fat, or cartilage, along with various other soft tissues. Sarcomas originate in mesenchymal connective tissues or the embryonic mesodermal tissues found in muscle, bone, fat, or cartilage.

The formation of the term has specific meaning. The prefix (sarco-) comes from the Greek word "sarkos," meaning "flesh." The suffix (-oma) also comes from the Greek and means "swelling" or "tumor." The suffix, -oma, is typically used to refer to a benign tumor. Thus, the term fibroma refers to a benign tumor that has its starting point in the fibers of muscle or

Copyright © Mometrix Media. You have been licensed one copy of this document for personal use only. Any other reproduction or redistribution is strictly prohibited. All rights reserved.

nerves. Unfortunately, however, some tumorous growths that are cancerous also use the suffix -oma. Therefore, a chondrosarcoma refers to a malignant tumor that originates in the cartilage, and sarcoma refers more generally to any cancer of connective tissue. Other malignant tumors ending in the suffix -oma include melanoma, insulinoma, seminoma, and thymoma.

Melanoma

Melanoma is a malignant tumor or cancer that may or may not be accompanied by a dark pigmentation (if pigmented, it is usually black). This type of cancer is more commonly found in dogs than in cats. Melanoma can be unrelenting, and it often grows quickly. The tumor can metastasize or spread within the body quite rapidly. The spreading of this cancer occurs when the original tumor is transported by the lymphatic system to the lymph nodes or via the vascular system in blood cells. Dogs have a 1 in 20 chance of having any tumor diagnosed as malignant melanoma. The most common sites for development of melanoma are on the skin, on the animal's digits, and in the mouth (more particularly found on the face, trunk, feet, and scrotum). Animals with malignant melanoma are generally older, frequently 9 to 12 years of age. The tumor may have produced ulcers or bleeding. This form of cancer responds best to early detection and treatments. The chances for metastatic spread are increased with late detection of the cancer. Often, late detection will have given the cancer time to spread to various bodily organs. The late diagnosis of malignant melanoma may preclude successful treatment. Certainly the prognosis is never as good as it could have been with earlier detection. Late-staged melanoma is not treatable with chemotherapy or radiation. The animal can be expected to survive for 2 to 3 months when the cancer reaches its most advanced stages.

Squamous cell carcinoma

Both cats and dogs can be diagnosed with squamous cell carcinoma. This is the most common type of malignant tumor that can develop in the epithelial layer of the skin, but it can also develop in the mucous membranes. This type of cancer is primarily found in cats, but it can also occur in dogs. It attacks the adjacent tissue and can spread to destroy bone in the animal's skeletal structure. The tumor appears grayish white or pink. It has an abnormally shaped mass. It is most often located in the gingiva, tonsils, and nose. Ulceration is associated with this cancer. Squamous cell carcinoma is aggressive but treatable. The veterinarian may apply surgery, radiation, or hyperthermia in the removal of the tumor.

Fibrosarcoma

Fibrosarcoma is the third most common cancerous tumor found in dogs. This cancer can quickly develop, and it has a tendency to spread. The tumor has an abnormal formation which presents as a firm nodule. Tumor-induced ulcerations and/or necrosis can sometimes also appear. The veterinarian will need to perform a biopsy before being able to make a clear diagnosis. However, the veterinarian may well give the caretaker a guarded prognosis once the diagnosis of fibrosarcoma has been determined. The veterinarian will surgically resect (remove) the cancerous tumor. However, it should be expected that a large mass of surrounding muscle and bone will also require removal. In addition, the patient will more than likely require follow-up treatment with chemotherapy and radiation.

Epulis

Not all tumors are malignant. One type of nonmalignant tumor is known as epulis. This oral tumor can be found in dogs and, rarely, in cats. Epulis is a non-malignant cancer that begins along the periodontal ligament. It will attack the adjacent tissue and spread to the bone. There are 3 kinds of epulides: fibromatous, ossifying, and acanthomatous. Fibromatous epulides are fashioned from a resilient tissue fiber. Ossifying epulides are fashioned from bone cells and fibrous tissue. The Ossifying tumor can develop into cancer. Acanthomatous epulides are detrimental to the bone structure. They are extensively intrusive and will infiltrate (grow into) normal bone. Once it has engulfed the bone it will destroy it. The animal may exhibit drooling, loss of appetite, difficulty eating, and bad breath. The tumor may also be of a size and located in such a way as to cause the animal difficulty in breathing.

Therapy

It is often possible to entirely remove a tumor through a surgical procedure, particularly when it is both localized and encapsulated. It is important to note that malignant tumors should be removed along with approximately 2 to 3 cm or 1 to 2 inches of healthy tissue bordering the tumor. One type of surgery known as cryosurgery is done by freezing tiny external epithelial lesions with liquid nitrogen or N2O. The cancerous tissue is thereby frozen, following which it dies and can be sloughed off, débrided, or otherwise removed. Another procedure, known as chemotherapy, applies cytotoxic agents to the cancerous regions. Chemotherapy cannot be described as a cure-all for cancer, as it is toxic not only to cancer cells but to healthy cells as well. However, chemotherapy has been able to create a state of remission in some patients. The types of cancers which best respond to this type of treatment are known as systemic and metastatic cancers.

Cytotoxic agents are capable of destroying neoplastic cells, primarily by disrupting nucleic acid and protein synthesis. Cytotoxic agents (often referred to as chemotherapy medications) are toxic to all cells, but tend to be taken up faster by cells that are rapidly dividing — a characteristic common to cancer cells. Because bone marrow cells also divide rapidly, patients often become immunosuppressed when cytotoxic agents delay the production of crucial blood and immunological cells. Common side effects of chemotherapy include alopecia, cardiotoxicity, vomiting, diarrhea, pancreatitis, hepatosis, neutropenia, thrombocytopenia, anemia, neurotoxicity, and renal toxicity. Staff should wear protective garments to reduce harmful side effects induced by even incidental contact with powerful cytotoxic agents. Recommended garments include latex gloves, long-sleeved lab coats or long-sleeved surgical gowns, and safety goggles. The sleeves on the garments should have close-fitting cuffs. In addition, the waste products must be discarded according to specific biomedical waste guidelines. This waste includes syringes, IV administration sets, gauze, and gloves. The waste should be discarded in a plastic bag that has been securely closed.

Another procedure known as radiotherapy applies a dose of ionizing radiation to the cancerous region. Radiography interrupts the cell's DNA replication, which results in its death. Yet another technique is known as cauterization. This technique uses various methods to burn away tiny epithelial tumors.

Physical examination of ruminants

A veterinarian can glean considerable useful information by taking a few moments to observe an animal from outside its enclosure. The veterinarian should take stock of the condition of the animal's eyes, stance and carriage, the body tone, movement and gait, as well as urine and manure output. In addition, the veterinarian should ascertain and document how much food and water is being consumed by the animal. There should be a specific set of procedures applied to every physical examination to ensure that it is thorough and complete. These procedures will produce consistent results for each patient examined. Typically, the procedures flow forward from the originating point of the examination, which should begin at the animal's nose. The examination should then move from the head of the animal down to the tail, with attention paid to intervening areas of the patient. The veterinarian should use a stethoscope to listen to the sounds coming from the animal's heart, lungs, and abdomen. The condition of the animal's skin, coat, mane, tail, and hooves should also be observed and recorded.

Thorough documentation is important. A complete recording should include all abrasions, swellings, and discharges emanating from the patient. The veterinarian should record the animal's temperature, pulse, and respiration (or TPR). The stethoscope is applied to the left paralumbar fossa to pick up any sounds emanating from rumen contractions. The ribs, vertebral column, and pelvis should be palpated (i.e., examined by touch) with a gentle pressure. This helps the veterinarian determine if the animal is suffering from areas of sensitivity, and to check for malnourishment by detecting the musculature and adipose layers of the animal.

The balling gun is a plastic or metal instrument used to give a ruminant animal an oral medication or vitamin dosage. The animal's head should be immobile when the balling gun is applied. The animal will be forced to open its mouth when the bridge of its nose is held. Stress should be directed to the hard palate. The balling gun is then inserted into the opening. The oral dosage is directed to the base of the patient's tongue. The jaws of a swine are held ajar with a bar speculum. The boluses or capsules can then be inserted at the base of the tongue by utilizing the balling gun.

Veins for samples and drug administration

Cattle
The jugular vein is the ideal spot to administer large amounts of fluids and/or medications to an animal. This spot can also be utilized to take venous blood samples from the animal. The animal's head is held immobile through the use of a head catch device. The device should be pulled in an upward direction towards the opposite side of the animal. The syringe must be of adequate size (measured in mL or cc) for the liquid being injected. The needle used usually ranges from 16 to 18 gauge (the smaller the number the larger the bore) and 1 to 3 inches in length.

The vein in the tail is ideal for smaller quantities of fluid. Smaller animals should be held securely in place by bending the tail straight forward from its base. The animal will not be able to make a movement to the left or to the right when this hold is firmly applied. The syringe must be of adequate size for the liquid being injected, with a needle that ranges in bore diameter from 18 to 20 gauge and about 1 to 1.5 inches in length. A smaller size syringe is applicable for the administration of more modest amounts of fluid. Another spot that can be employed for injections is the milk vein. However, this vein does have a tendency to form hematomas when stress is applied. The needle used with this vein is frequently 14 gauge and 2 to 3 inches in length.

Pigs
Swine should be given large quantities of intravenous liquid through the cranial vena cava. The mature swine requires use of an 18 to 20 gauge needle, 3 to 4 inches in length. This is comparable in length to a 7.5 to 10 cm needle. The jugular fossa closest to the manubrium sterni of the pig can be employed as a guide to ensure proper placement or alignment into the cranial vena cava. The needle must be inserted in a perpendicular direction towards the neck facing the left shoulder.

The ear artery is known as the caudal auricular artery. This artery is ideal for giving the pig smaller quantities of liquid. The syringe should be inserted with gentle pressure. The syringe must be of adequate size for the liquid being injected. The needle used usually ranges from 18 to 22 gauge and 1 to 1.5 inches in length. This needle is comparable to a 2.5 to 3.75 cm needle length. Intravenous administrations within the vein typically require the use of a 19 to 21 gauge butterfly needle.

Intramuscular injections

Cattle
Cattle can receive intramuscular injections through the lateral cervical muscles of the body. Mature cattle will receive injections with a 16, 18, or 20 gauge needle that is 1.5 to 2 inches in length. It is comparable to a 3.75 to 5 cm needle. Only 15 to 20 mL of medication can be administered at each specific intramuscular (IM) injection site. Smaller-sized calves may require smaller-sized needles. The smaller-sized needles can be used to administer 10 to 15 mL of medication into an animal.

The area should be desensitized with a couple of modest taps from the flat side of the hand in a balled up position with fingers closed (i.e., a half-fist). This will also give the animal an opportunity to steady itself before the needle is inserted. The best way to apply the intramuscular injection is to align the needle in the proper position before attaching the syringe. The medication can then be introduced into the patient with this intramuscular injection.

Sheep, goats, and pigs
Sheep and goats can receive an intramuscular injection through the lateral cervical muscles. Mature sheep and goats will receive injections with a needle ranging from 18 to 20 gauge and

1.5 inches in length (comparable to a 3.75 cm needle). Smaller sized animals will need a 20 to 22 gauge needle. The maximum capacity of medication intramuscularly given to an adult-sized animal is 15 mL. The normal quantity typically measures about 5 to 10 mL.

Swine are given the injection through the dorsolateral neck muscles. This site is deemed to be the most appropriate for pigs. The pig will require an 18 to 20 gauge needle that is about 1.5 inches in length (comparable to a 3.75 cm needle). This is an appropriate size for a mature pig. The maximum amount of fluids appropriately given intramuscularly is 1 to 15 mL, depending upon the size of the animal and the area injected.

Subcutaneous injections

Subcutaneous injections for cattle are administered in site regions from the cranial area to the shoulder and lateral to the animal's neckline. The ideal needle bore will range from 16 to 18 gauge, with a 1.5 inch or 3.75 cm needle length. The veterinarian can use his or her discretion to establish the volume of the injection. However, it is best that adult cattle only receive about 250 mL/site, at most. Younger cattle should receive a maximum of about 50 mL/site.

Smaller ruminants will be given an injection along the cranial to the shoulder region. This injection is given in a lateral direction from the neck. The animal should only receive about 5 mL of fluid per site. The recommended needle bore ranges from 18 to 20 gauge, with a 1 inch or 2.5 cm needle length. The injection is given at the lateral side of the neck near the base of the pig's ear, with 1 to 3 mL injected per site. The maximum amount is dependent upon the size of the pig. The recommended needle bore ranges from 16 to 18 gauge with a 1 to 1.5 inch needle. This is comparable to a 2.5 to 3.75 cm needle.

Milk sample for bacterial culture

The identification and treatment of mastitis is critical to an animal's good physical condition. Mastitis is inflammation of the animal's udder. This condition can have particularly detrimental effects upon a dairy herd. The dairy herd will have a sample of its milk taken for a culture. The samples are first tested for a simple positive or negative result, as this screening reduces the costs associated with more detailed laboratory testing. Any positive test result will indicate the need for further, more definitive testing. The samples should be collected from the animals before the milking process begins. However, samples may also be collected from an animal after milking has been completed, during the 6 or more hours that follow the prior milking episode.

In taking a sample, the udder should be thoroughly cleansed. Each teat should be wiped with alcohol beginning from the farthest point to the nearest in proximity. Then the teat should air dry. The initial milk stream must be thrown out. The midstream milk is collected and saved for the sample. The milk stream is aimed in a straight line towards the sample vial.

Horses

Temperature and pulse

A mature, fully grown horse has a normal body temperature between 37 to 38.5 °C (between 98.6 to 101.3 °F). The normal pulse rate is in the range of 28 to 45 beats per minute. The veterinarian can auscultate, or listen to, the horse's heart with a stethoscope. When doing so, the veterinarian may well hear only 2-3 specific heart sounds. However, there are times that more than 3 are heard. The full array of 4 can be notated according to the phases of the cardiac cycle, as depicted by the symbols S1, S2, S3, and S4. The most prominent sound is normally associated with ventricular contraction. This sound is depicted by the symbol S1. The second sound that the animal will display is associated with the semilunar valves closing. This second sound is depicted by the symbol S2. The third sound that the animal will display is associated with the blood rushing into the ventricles. This faint sound is depicted by the symbol S3. The fourth sound, rarely heard, is associated with atrial contraction. This fourth sound is depicted by the symbol S4.

Cardiac rhythm

The mature horse has a number of heart rhythms that can fall within the normal range. A thorough examination should be completed and all of the following cardiac performance indices and measures should be recorded: heart rate, rhythm, intensity, any deficiency or absence of standard sounds, and any unusual sounds — all of which can be classified as cardiac arrhythmias (sometimes referred to as dysrhythmias). Two of the more common and prominent abnormal rhythms in the heart are tachycardia and bradycardia. Tachycardia is a sustained overly-rapid heart rate. This is defined (in a horse) as a heart rate of more than 50 beats per minute. Bradycardia is an unusually slow heart rate. This is defined (in a horse) as a heart rate that is lower than 20 beats per minute. Irregular beats, skipped beats, incomplete beats, etc, are often associated with both of these forms of arrhythmias. The condition known as hypocalcemia can result in brachycardia. Hypocalcemia is a condition where the animal has an extremely low level of calcium present in the blood.

Atrioventricular blocks

The term atrioventricular block is abbreviated as AV block. This condition occurs when the atrial depolarization is not relayed to the ventricles, or when there is an unduly prolonged delay between atrial depolarization and ventricular depolarization. There are 3 recognized degrees of AV block. First-degree AV block is characterized by a lengthened PR interval, arising from dysfunction of the AV node. There are few symptoms or problems associated with this degree of AV block. In second-degree AV block, one or more (but not all) of the atrial impulses fail to communicate on to the ventricles. While few patients show symptoms, those who do may experience fainting and dizziness. In third-degree AV block (sometimes referred to as "complete" heart block), no atrial impulses (sometimes called supraventricular impulses) are relayed to the ventricles. This leaves the ventricles to generate a rhythm from alternate conduction sites (often septally derived). In an electrocardiograph, the P wave and the QRS complex can be seen to function independently from each other. These factors will be used to establish the presence of a complete heart block. Some horses with second-degree heart block may be in poor health. However, a horse with second-degree heart block may or may not be diagnosed with a heart disease.

Normal respiration

The normal respiration or breathing rhythm for a mature horse is 8 to 20 breaths per minute. The veterinarian will make a careful observation of the horse's flanks and nostrils in observing respiratory function. In addition, the veterinarian will use a stethoscope positioned on the trachea and in the left and right lung fields to listen to the passage of air during inspiration and expiration. In this process the veterinarian is trying to find evidence of sounds associated with abnormal respiration.

The normal respiration rhythm of the horse has a consistent pattern: 1) a pause; 2) followed by inspiration or breathing inwards; and 3) expiration or breathing out. Horses that are in an excited condition can exhibit deeper inspiratory breaths than expiratory breaths (i.e., gasping, etc). This can be seen in an abnormal respiration rhythm. Further, strenuous exercise may bring on the following: coughing, nasal discharge, epistaxis (nose bleeds), hyperpnea (abnormally deep or rapid breathing), and dyspnea (difficult or labored breathing). These symptoms can indicate that the animal has a respiratory condition. The horse should next receive an endoscopy. This test will be beneficial in helping the veterinarian to determine the condition of the horse's pharynx and trachea.

Injections

Intravenous
The animal receiving an intravenous injection should have the injection site cleansed to prevent infection and to destroy disease-carrying microorganisms. This can be accomplished by using a cotton ball doused in alcohol and firmly swabbing the injection site. The horse's jugular vein is a prominent vessel that meets the criteria for an injection site. However, there are times when other sites may be more appropriate. Alternate sites include the thoracic, cephalic, and saphenous veins.

An IV injection is an effective way to administer a fast-acting drug. An IV route can also be used to introduce sizeable quantities of fluid into the animal's body. In addition, an IV site can be used when blood is collected from the animal. The veterinarian can be assured that an injection has been correctly administered into the vein when blood can be drawn back through the needle or catheter.

The aspiration or suction of fluids or gases from the body can be accomplished with a syringe. An indwelling catheter used for these purposes can be fastened into place with a sewing technique or glue. The site should be further protected with an overlay of tape and Elastoplast for added hygienic protection and security.

Intramuscular
The animal receiving an intramuscular (IM) injection should have the injection site cleansed to prevent infection from occurring. This is accomplished by using a cotton ball doused in alcohol and firmly swabbing the injection site. Some likely places for an intramuscular injection are in the muscles of the neck, the semitendinosus muscle (in the thigh), the gluteus muscle (in the flank), and the pectoralis descendens (a chest muscle). The medical staff should be careful to avoid injections near joints, blood vessels, or large fat deposits. The effectiveness (in duration) of some drugs can be extended with the application of an IM injection.

It is also important to note that some drugs require administration into the body through intramuscular injections alone. For instance, an injection of procaine penicillin directly into the bloodstream will result in a harmful reaction in the patient. The severity of the reaction is usually directly related to the time that it takes for the reaction to take place. Acute reactions can be produced instantaneously. However, a longer period of time may elapse before evidence of a milder reaction appears. The medical staff should be on the alert for the following reactions: restlessness, agitation, head tossing, snorting, eye rolling, violent thrashing, or a state of collapse.

Routine vaccinations

There are routine sets of vaccinations that should be administered to horse based upon geographical location. The prevalence of a particular disease can relate directly to the region in which the animal resides. Animals in the United States should be given the following vaccinations: Eastern and Western encephalomyelitis, tetanus, and influenza. Young horses should also receive the vaccination known as rhinopneumonitis. Some locations also recommend the administration of the vaccination known as the Strangles vaccine. Use of this vaccination is becoming more widespread. In addition, the intranasal administration of many vaccines is also increasing. It is a common occurrence to vaccinate an animal for rabies regardless of the geographic location. Revised vaccination protocols have increased the prevalence of the West Nile virus and Potomac horse fever vaccines. These vaccinations should now be given to horses in areas that are both high and low risk.

Horses located in the Ontario, Canada region should be given the following vaccinations: rabies, tetanus, Rhinopneumonitis or EHV-4/1, and West Nile virus. Horses that travel outside of the region will be given the following vaccinations: Eastern and Western encephalomyelitis, Strangles, and Potomac horse fever or equine monocytic ehrlichiosis.

Gastrointestinal ailments

Gastrointestinal ailments in horses can be attributed to a number of possible problems. These problems include overfeeding, parasites, twisted intestines, defective feed, an irregular feeding schedule, and sudden changes in feed. The animal exhibiting the following clinical signs could be suffering from a gastrointestinal ailment: restlessness, getting up and down frequently, agitation, hoof pawing, persistently pacing the stall or confinement area, rolling,

- 29 -

biting at, or persistently watching their flank, and kicking at the abdominal region. Other bodily symptoms include: a distended abdomen, sweating, grinding teeth, increased heart and respiration rates, increased CRT (capillary refill time, usually in the gingival area), and diminished appetite. The animal's mucous membranes and gums should be checked. The gums can have a visible red or blue toxic line located right above the horse's teeth. The mucous membranes can change to a pale, bright brick red or bluish color. Cyanosis is indicated by a bluish color, and means there is not enough oxygen in the horse's bloodstream. The following conditions may also be present: hypermotility, hypomotility, or the entire absence of gastrointestinal motility. The horse may even sit in a stance like a dog or with its legs extended out in a sawhorse-like posture.

Colic
Colic can cause a horse to experience considerable pain in the abdominal region, and is the number one cause of premature equine fatality. This common problem can be a result of the following: poor feed or feeding and hydration patterns; intestinal tears, displacements, torsions, or hernias; disproportionate gas; sporadic cramps; ileus; parasitic infections; volvulus; intussusception; impactions; obstructions; displacement; inguinal hernias; or ulcers. The colic's degree of severity may not be readily evident depending upon the disposition of the horse. Therefore, careful observation is recommended. In addition, the horse can be placed on a treatment regimen involving the following: fluid therapy, anti-inflammatory drugs, mineral oil, anti-flatulence medication, and anti-ulcer medication. Intestinal injuries (tears, torsions, hernias, etc) typically require corrective surgery. The horse will need the following checked: vital signs, motility, and fecal output. The horse's state of hydration may be observed when a nasogastric tube is passed and gastrointestinal reflux is achieved. The horse will require regular moderate exercise, typically by being walked. The animal should be reintroduced to food slowly and gradually to reduce upset in the animal's digestive system.

Colitis
Acute colitis is a condition that has yet to be fully understood. The exact cause of the disease is still a mystery. However, it appears some animals may develop colitis due to the following: dietary changes, excessive consumption of carbohydrates, Clostridium perfringens or colitis X, Clostridium difficile, Potomac horse fever, antibiotic therapy, and the overuse of NSAIDs. Acute colitis may be present in the horse that exhibits the following signs and symptoms: inappetence, listlessness, depression, abdominal pain, hyper- or hypomotile gastric motility, increased heart and respiration rates, discolored mucous membranes, increased CRT (capillary refill time), diarrhea, dehydration, hypoproteinemia, imbalance of electrolytes, metabolic acidosis, and shock. Shock, in this situation, can often be attributed to endotoxemia (caused by endotoxin molecules released during the rapid growth or death of gram-negative bacteria). Mucous membranes that have a brick or dark red color, or else a muddy or bluish or cyanotic coloration, can be associated with acute colitis. The animal should be treated with fluid therapy, consisting of a balanced electrolyte solution.

A horse with colitis should be treated with fluid therapy. This should reduce the inflammation and spasms experienced by the horse in the colon and abdominal region. The fluid therapy should consist of a balanced electrolyte solution. Sometimes adequate amounts of potassium, chloride, and calcium are missing from the animal's diet. This can be corrected via supplementation during fluid therapy. Fluid therapy can also be used for the correction of metabolic acidosis. Metabolic acidosis is caused by an increase in the acidity of the blood. The result is a low blood pH level. The correction is made by adding sodium bicarbonate or anti-inflammatory drugs to the fluid therapy administered to the animal. However, a plasma transfusion is required when the total protein is low. A vasodilator is an agent that opens and expands the blood vessels. This agent can be effective in combating the natural tendency toward vasoconstriction found in the equine medial and lateral digital arteries (located between the hoof wall and the distal phalanx). One commonly used vasodilator is known as nitroglycerin.

Salmonellosis
Many horses with diarrhea are diagnosed with salmonellosis. Salmonellosis is the number one cause of infectious diarrhea in horses for at least 2 reasons. First, salmonella is a zoonotic organism (can be passed from animals to humans) that is essentially ubiquitous in the equine environment (up to 20% of all horses may "shed" the organism, as it is present in their natural intestinal flora). Second, it is extremely contagious to other equines. Therefore, this contagious disease must be managed very carefully. Salmonellosis can also be triggered by stress in the animal. Some causes for a significant degree of stress are evident in the following: animals transported in a trailer, sudden changes in feeding, use of antibiotics, sickness, surgery, or immunosuppression. It is important for signs of the disease not to be mistaken for similar signs displayed in animals with colitis. The animal can also have an acute case of diarrhea. Notably, the consistency and categorization of the diarrhea is profuse, watery, and foul-smelling. The animal may have pyrexia (a fever), and may also show signs of anorexia.

In the event infectious Salmonellosis is discovered, the animal should be isolated and only one handler should treat the animal to reduce cross-contamination risks. The handler should wear a gown, gloves, and protective boot covers. Hand washing with a bactericidal solution is essential. Boots worn in the isolated horse's stall must be washed in a foot bath. Fluid therapy is given using a balanced electrolyte solution to reduce chances for dehydration and electrolyte disorders. Animals with hypoproteinemia may well need a plasma transfusion. The animal's vital signs must be taken at regular intervals to ensure that the body is functioning adequately. The horse can be fed as often as its appetite allows. However, grain is not included in the diet during this time.

Intestinal clostridial infections
Intestinal clostridial infections cause severe inflammation of the intestines. Colitis X, a widespread form of this disease, is usually discovered only after the death of the animal (during a postmortem examination). It is similar to colitis. Diarrhea is not observed in its early stages. Chronic pain is generated in the abdominal region within hours of contracting the disease. Hypermotility is typically seen. It is treated with an oral dose of antibiotics such as bacitracin. This disease should be treated in largely the same manner as that of colitis or salmonellosis.

Potomac horse fever

Potomac horse fever is abbreviated as PHF. It is also known as monocytic ehrlichiosis. One common vector implicated in spreading the infective organism, Ehrlichia risticii, is through snails. In the northeastern United States a peak season exists for the spreading of this disease, largely between the months of June through August. Signs of the disease include depression, anorexia, and pyrexia; a decrease in sounds in the gut; abdominal pain; and diarrhea. Treatments involve: a) isolation of the animal; b) oxytetracycline; c) fluid therapy consisting of a balanced electrolytic solution; and d) frequent monitoring of vital signs. Laminitis is a serious concern. Vaccines preventing PHF have a high rate of effectiveness, but are not totally foolproof.

Anterior enteritis

Anterior enteritis can be linked to Clostridium spp (i.e., including multiple subspecies). However, this disease is normally thought of as idiopathic, with no apparent or known source. Clinical symptoms of this disease involve the following: severe colic, higher heart and respiration rates, and a probability of pyrexia (fever). Horses are unable to expel excess stomach contents by way of emesis (vomiting). Thus, the treatment of anterior enteritis involves insertion of a nasogastric tube (NG tube). This tube is used to collect any gastric reflux fluids and to relieve gastric and intestinal fluid distension. Without placement of this tube, outright gastric rupture may occur from fluid overload. If the patient exhibits a lessening in symptoms after the NG tube is placed, then it is highly probable that the patient does not have an intestinal obstruction and it is more likely that the patient has anterior enteritis. Anterior enteritis often is mistaken for an obstructed bowel. A rectal exam is needed for verification purposes and to make a more conclusive (albeit not always definitive) diagnosis.

Fluid therapy provides replacement of essential fluids, as oral fluid intake is trapped by the enteritis. A jugular vein access is usually needed, as the animal may require as much as 60 to 100 liters (30 to 50 gallons) of replacement fluids daily. The horse requires the monitoring of these vital signs: temperature, color of mucous membranes, CRT (capillary refill time) in the gingival area, and digital pulses. Toxemia can occur as a result of the bacterial toxins present in the horse's bloodstream. This poisonous condition can be a direct result of the severe intestinal upset that accompanies anterior enteritis.

Hyperkalemic periodic paralysis

Genetic mutations can cause some diseases to occur in animals. Some Quarter Horse sires have a particular genetic mutation that brings about the disease known as hyperkalemic periodic paralysis. Hyperkalemic periodic paralysis can be abbreviated as HYPP. This disease has the following clinical symptoms: muscle fasciculations; incidences of colic, sweating, respiratory distress, and a prolapsed third eyelid (the nictitating membrane which lies on the inside corner of the eye and closes diagonally over it); loose feces; and ataxia (unsteady gait). A blood test can be used to reveal if the horse is a homozygous affected animal, with 2

- 32 -

identical genes. Or, the test may reveal that the horse is a heterozygous carrier with genetic variants. Ideally, however, the test will reveal that the horse has a normal genetic makeup. Breeding is not recommended for horses that have a positive blood test. In addition, horses that have HYPP should not be ridden, as gait and balance issues can present a danger to both the animal and the rider. The horse should be given a low potassium diet, and lots of fresh water. It is best not to give the horse alfalfa hay, feeding grass, or oat hay. In addition, stress should be reduced as much as possible.

Tetanus

The bacteria known as Clostridium tetani can be found in some soils. This bacterium is responsible for the infection known as tetanus or "lockjaw." The bacterium typically enters the body through a puncture wound. The neurotoxins created by the clostridium tetani are able to severely impact the nervous system. The horse shows the following symptoms: a) muscle stiffness as evidenced in a sawhorse stance; b) a decrease in water and feed consumption; c) hypersensitivity to light and noise; and d) muscle fasciculations. The horse that has tetanus should receive a tetanus antitoxin booster. This booster is beneficial in binding the circulating tetanus toxins to the antitoxin in the vaccine. The puncture wound requires cleansing. In addition, any excess fluids around the site should be drained off. Topical penicillin is rubbed onto the injury. The animal should be given an IV infusion with penicillin and other fluids. It is recommended that horses receive an annual tetanus vaccination. This cuts down on the likelihood that an animal will contract the infection at a later date.

Rabies

Rabies is a result of a virus known as rhabdovirus. This virus works to damage the central nervous system. The bite of an infected animal allows the transmission of the disease to another animal. The infected animal's saliva is an infective source of the rhabdovirus. This virus can also be transmitted through any open wound or through the mucous membranes. Some infected animals will exhibit high levels of aggression. Other symptoms include dysphagia, hydrophobia, and self-inflicted wounds. If the handler suspects that a horse has rabies, the horse should be immediately isolated. The handler should protect himself by wearing the appropriate clothing, including gloves and other protective gear. Rabies can be transmitted to the handler, as it is a virus with zoonotic (animal to human transmission) potential. This high potential, in conjunction with the lack of a cure for rabies, results in a rabid horse's euthanasia. Since rabies can only be positively identified through a postmortem examination, it becomes necessary to also euthanize animals that are suspected of having rabies. The best medical advice is to make sure that the animal receives its annual vaccination.

EHV-1

The acronym for Equine Herpes Virus 1 is EHV-1. This viral rhinopneumonitis is an organism that primarily infects the respiratory system and endothelial tissues, but which is capable of attacking the nervous system as well. Typical infective symptoms include: fever, depression, inappetence, nasal discharge, and a cough. However, if neurologically afflicted, the horse can exhibit the following symptoms: ungainly movements, incontinence, posterior ataxia (lack of muscle control in the hind limbs), and an absence of tail tone. The horse may be found sitting as a dog or in a recumbent position. This is attributed to the paralytic state of the animal's hind legs. The infected expectant mother may spontaneously abort an unborn fetus.

To reduce fetal risks, the animal should be given a vaccination in the 5th, 7th, and 9th month of the pregnancy. The vaccine is Pneumabort K +1b. Abortion does not necessarily have to occur if the animal is infected during later gestational periods. Harm to the foal in utero is evident when a stillbirth foal is delivered. A live foal may also die shortly after delivery. The horse may be given antibiotics, anti-inflammatory drugs, or corticosteroids. It is recommended that horses receive a preventive vaccination. However, abortions or neurological diseases can still occur if the vaccination does not provide enough protection.

Strangles

The bacteria Streptococcus equi (S. equi subsp. equi) is a gram-positive coccus that can harm the infected horse's upper respiratory system. The bacteria produce the condition known as Strangles. This condition causes the horse to experience a number of problems associated with breathing and swallowing. This is a highly contagious disease that requires the animal to be placed in isolation. The horse suffering with Strangles will have significant swelling in the lymph nodes, particularly those located underneath the mandible, the guttural pouches, and in the throat. Over time, the lymph nodes develop into empyema abscesses (pus-filled lesions). The horse should receive hot packs on these swellings. The hot packs facilitate the abscesses opening and draining. In addition, many of the abscesses may require lancing to allow the excess fluid to drain. During this time the infected horse may experience dysphagia, finding it difficult to swallow. If this happens, the horse should be given additional fluids. The infected horse should also be fed slurries, which are a liquified mixture of water and feed.

The animal infected with Strangles requires liberal, readily available amounts of fresh water. The infected horse should be kept warm and dry. The horse should also be given antipyretics and antibiotics. An antipyretic is a drug to reduce the animal's fever. Antibiotics are beneficial in destroying the virulent bacteria in the body. However, this highly contagious disease must still be carefully monitored. All materials that come into contact with the sick animal should be disposed of by fire or disinfected thoroughly. This disease does not have a vaccination that can entirely halt its progression. However, the vaccine that is available has been proven to reduce the seriousness of the symptoms associated with the disease. Vaccines should be given to the horse by way of an intranasal administration (through the nose of the animal).

EHV-4

The acronym for Equine Herpes Virus 4 is EHV-4. This virus produces a rhinopneumonitis, and is common throughout the globe. However, its infectious patterns differ significantly

- 34 -

from those common to EHV-1. Although EHV-1 also affects the respiratory tract and lymph nodes, it is predisposed to infecting endothelial tissue in the nose, lungs, adrenal glands, thyroid, and central nervous system. Thus, neurological problems and spontaneous abortions in gravid horses may also occur. By contrast, EHV-4 infections are largely localized to the respiratory tract and associated lymph glands, without these neurological and pregnancy issues.

EHV-4 is spread through close contact or through aerosolized body fluids (i.e., droplets scattered when sneezing, etc). This viral disease targets the horse's upper respiratory system, and causes increased respiratory symptoms such as wheezing, rhonchi, rales, and stridor. In addition, the lymph nodes will swell from the infection. It is highly recommended that the horse be placed in isolation, as there is a significant danger of cross-contamination. The horse's environment should be protected against undue cold and be well ventilated. The horse should be placed in a stall that is quiet, and should not be placed under stress. The animal will require brief periods of exercise, as this is beneficial to blood circulation and lymph systems. This disease cannot be totally prevented by preemptive vaccination, but post-infection vaccination is thought to reduce the seriousness of the associated symptoms.

EIA

The acronym for the Equine Infectious Anemia virus is EIA. Another name for this condition is Swamp Fever. This virus can be found in an animal's blood and semen. Transmission of the disease occurs primarily through blood, spread by biting flies (arthropods) and other blood-feeding insects. However, the animal can also contract this virus through blood transfusions and unsanitary needles used in various medical treatments. Finally, the disease can also be spread through semen, infecting mares and (because it can penetrate the placental barrier) their young. Infection is for life, with periods of remission and exacerbation recurring in due course. Infected horses will have the following symptoms: pyrexia (fever), depression, weight loss, anorexia, and anemia. All infected horses are carriers of this disease even when they display no symptoms. The animal with this disease should be euthanized. In each state or province, local, state, provincial, and federal regulations should be consulted regarding the laws concerning euthanasia. Horses that are not put to sleep should be placed in isolation to prevent further contamination of other animals. This isolation must last the length of the horse's lifespan, as there is no known cure for Swamp Fever or EIA. Total isolation (including insect-free isolation) is the only way to keep other horses from contracting the disease.

Laminitis

The disease known as laminitis impacts a horse's feet. This disease causes the laminae or protective plate inside the horse's hoof to become swollen and irritated. This inflammation is usually experienced more in the front hoofs of a horse than in the hind hoofs. However, there are occasions when the hoofs in the hind quarters will also become inflamed. Laminitis can result from the following: overconsumption of grain, ingesting too much cold water, endotoxemia, concussion, hormonal influences, aftermath of a viral respiratory disease, aftermath of a drug treatment, and overeating in lavish pastures. Horses with this condition display a lack of motivation and energy. Some horses display apprehension. Other symptoms include pyrexia, depression, lack of appetite, and sensitivity when hoof testing is conducted (typically by way of a manually operated device that tests for pressure-sensitive points on a horse's feet). Horses with laminitis will exhibit an irregular gait characterized by toe pointing and rocking onto the heel. This gait relieves pressure on the tender area of the toe. The hoof wall will also be hotter to the touch than is normally experienced.

With the hoof disease laminitis, the heat felt in the hoof wall is the result of increased in blood flow in that area. The digital pulses will also be out of the normal range. In acute cases, the coffin bone will rotate and penetrate the sole of the horse's foot. A radiograph can detect the extent of the rotation. Treatment includes anti-inflammatory drugs, acepromazine, fluids such as LRS (lactated Ringer's solution), and trimming the hoof in a restorative fashion. Vasodilators known as isoxsuprine hydrochloride and nitroglycerine can be applied to the horse's medial and lateral digital arteries. Vasodilators are medicines that can expand the blood vessels to lower blood pressure and ease the flow of blood. The horse should be given grass and hay to eat. Grains are not recommended. Cold hosing and icing the feet are treatments that have been applied by some veterinarians. However, others strongly disapprove of this practice.

Navicular syndrome

Navicular syndrome is not fully understood. The origin of the disease remains a mystery. However, the disease does produce a lameness and specific deterioration of the navicular bone (a small bone in a horse's foot). Horses suffering with navicular syndrome may display a variety of symptoms. These symptoms include stumbling, shorter strides, and periods where the horse goes lame. The horse's aversion to hoof testing may be attributed to the extreme amount of pain the horse is experiencing in the hoof region. Mechanical hoof testers cause considerable pain when pressure is applied to the sole of the foot of a horse with this disease. The horse that exhibits this reluctance should also be given the following tests: flexion tests, nerve blocking, and radiographs.

The horse can be treated with the following: anti-inflammatory medication, vasodilators, and corrective foot trimming and shoeing. One vasodilator often used for this condition is isoxsuprine hydrochloride. Some horses require a surgical neurectomy. This procedure is conducted along the nerve to the foot. The nerve is cut above the fetlock. However, this procedure should only be used when all other alternatives have been exhausted.

Radiographic examination

The procedures surrounding a radiographic examination primarily involve appropriate measures for the safe use of radiation. One standard view taken is with the horse standing with its leg directly underneath the plate. The technician will hold the plate parallel to the leg to obtain a proper radiographic view approximation. Other standard radiographs involve the following views: lateral, medial oblique, lateral oblique, anterior-posterior, flexed for the fetlock and carpus, and skyline of the carpus. Additional radiograph views may be obtained

- 36 -

with the horse standing on a cassette enclosed in a sturdy Plexiglas shield. This technique provides extra views of the feet. A portable unit is best applied in obtaining views of the feet, fetlocks, carpus, and hocks. The larger units (stationary and immobile due to size) are more efficient for obtaining views of the shoulder, stifle, and head regions. Radiographs of the pelvis are taken when the horse is in a dorsal recumbent position. However, the horse will need to be sedated with an anesthetic for this procedure to be carried out.

Nuclear scintigraphy

Nuclear scintigraphy is an imaging technique used to evaluate the kidneys, bones, thyroid gland, and brain. It requires that technetium (a radionuclide or radioactive isotope) be infused into the body with a syringe. The infusion is given to the horse by intravenous means. The animal will then be scanned to locate and track the radioactive isotope. The isotope appears as a radiographic "hot spot" approximately 2 hours after the injection has been given to the animal. The lower limbs of the animal should be scanned about 20 minutes after infusion of the isotope. The horse will be in a radioactive state for a period of 24 to 36 hours following the procedure. During this time the animal should be left alone except for feeding and watering. However, water should not be given to the animal whenever the pelvis is being examined, as the full bladder will obscure certain views of the pelvis. The veterinarian may give the horse a diuretic to reduce the size of the bladder. One example of a diuretic is Lasix, which may be administered parenterally.

Nuclear scintigraphy is an appropriate examination for tendon injuries, suspected suspensory injuries, and horses with a crippling injury or lameness. Of particular benefit is the ability to detect tibial stress fractures, condylar fractures, and pelvis, carpus, and hock injuries.

Diagnostic Imaging

X-rays

X-rays are derived from the energy produced by electrons or negatively charged particles within an atom. This energy is converted to electromagnetic radiation. The radiation produces energy particles known as photons. Photons do not have any mass or electrical charge, but they can carry electromagnetic (EM) energy. When EM-carrying photons crash into and pass through matter, the x-ray picture is created. An x-ray tube has filters that are able to direct the source of electrons at the object toward which it is aimed. The x-ray tube must have the following components: a source of electrons, a method to accelerate the electrons, a defined path, a target, and an encompassing envelope in which to create a vacuum. The electrode pair (a heated cathode and an anode carrying a powerful voltage charge) is the source from which the EM-charged photons are derived. The cathode is capable of releasing electrons when subjected to heat. The electrons are sped up when drawn toward the charged anode, and their collision with the anode produces EM-charged photons, which are aimed to produce a collision with the intended target. Approximately 99% of the energy created is heat and 1% is x-rays (photons carrying EM energy). EM energy is measured as a kilovoltage peak or potential kVp. This energy can be harnessed and adjusted in accordance with the specifications of the particular x-ray machine. The kVp of the electrons establishes the penetration strength of the x-rays.

X-ray tube

An x-ray tube consists of the following components: a cathode filament, an anode plate, a focusing cup, a target, a glass envelope (within which a vacuum is created), an aluminum filter, and a beryllium window. The x-ray tube generates the photons carrying the electromagnetic charge, and directs them along a targeted pathway. The cathode filament is usually made from tungsten. The tungsten filament is a coiled wire that releases electrons when heat is applied to its surface. The cathode filament is situated across from the focusing cup and the anode plate. The filament maintains a negative potential throughout the heating process. The electrons are drawn to the positively charged anode at great speed. The anode can be immobile or it can be put into a rotation. The target is described as tungsten with a copper stem. The target is fastened to the face of the anode. The entire x-ray device is encased within a tube-shaped Pyrex capsule that creates a vacuum. This is essential for x-ray generation. The x-rays are sent out through a small window fashioned from a thin section of glass. This glass absorbs a small quantity of x-rays or electromagnetic radiation.

X-ray machine

The x-ray machine must also include the following components: electrical circuits to control the x-ray tube, a control panel, and a tube stand. It has filters, collimators, and grids as part of its framework. The electrical circuits utilize high-voltage electricity to generate energy and speed. This speed allows the electrons to develop a high electromagnetic potential. The electrical circuits also supply a low-voltage electric current used for heating the cathode filament. A timer switch operates to measure exposure time in seconds. The rectification circuit is used to change the current supplied to the tube from alternating to direct current. The control panel is utilized to manage and regulate the kilovoltage peak, milliampere, milliampere-seconds, and/or seconds. This regulation is dependent upon the capacity of the x-ray machine. The kVp potential establishes the class of energy. The mA (milliampere) and involved time establishes the intensity of the x-rays. Kilovoltage peak is abbreviated as kVp. Milliampere is abbreviated as mA. Milliampere-seconds are abbreviated as mAs. The x-ray tube is set up on a foundation known as the tube stand.

Intensifying screens and screen speeds

The x-ray machine incorporates an intensifying screen made from a synthetic base covered in sheets of small luminescent phosphor crystals. These crystals function as a protective covering. Two intensifying screens are located on the interior fabric of the x-ray cassette. The film is packed in between these 2 screens. Visible light exposes the light-sensitive emulsion of the x-ray film when radiation connects with and illuminates the surface of the phosphor crystals. This is referred to as indirect imaging, and is responsible for more than 95% of the film's exposure to light. The screen functions to decrease the exposure time necessary to create a diagnostic image on film. Differences in intensifying screen speeds refer to the amount of exposure time required for the production of a diagnostic film. Screen speeds are measured as slow, medium, and fast. The best quality image is gained when slower speeds are used. Further, slower screen speeds do not have any significant problems relating to exposure times. Gradually, computerized x-ray machines are moving into the field. Relying on digital media, they are much more versatile to use, and they bypass the film development step altogether. Further, they have greater file-sharing and archival capacities. Thus, they are slowly replacing the older film and intensifying screen-based processes. In the interim, however, familiarity with traditional x-ray equipment remains important.

Fair to good resolutions can be obtained with medium-speed x-ray films. These require relatively low exposure times. Fast- speed films allow a more reduced exposure time and provide superior patient x-ray penetration. However, they trade speed for image quality. The poorer quality image is caused by the larger crystals and thicker layers applied in fast-speed screens. These blurred images show less detail than images taken with a medium or slow speed screen.

Characteristics of screen film

Film made with silver halide crystals or grains has a superior rate of sensitivity to the waves of light produced from the intensifying screens. This increased sensitivity allows a diagnostic radiograph to be created using a shorter exposure time. Greater resolution is obtained because of the finer image resolution grains on the film. This greater resolution is accomplished through longer exposure times. Shorter exposure times can only be achieved with larger grains on the films. The veterinarian will find that x-rays performed on animals

- 39 -

usually require only a medium-grain film. This medium- grain film is a concession made to obtain a reasonably good image resolution without an extended exposure time.

Characteristics of nonscreen film

Nonscreen x-ray film does not utilize intensifying screens. It has improved sensitivity to direct ionizing radiation. However, the nonscreen film will require a longer exposure time to work. Even so, it has the advantage of producing an image that has better detail-revealing resolution than that of an image gained via an intensifying screen. The film is packaged in a heavy envelope that does not allow light to pass through. This film is often used in dental offices, where the bulkiness of radiographic film coupled with an intensifying screen is prohibitive. The film speed is depicted by the label D or E. The faster nonscreen film speed is the E label.

Proper darkroom conditions

Proper darkroom conditions must also be maintained in clean, well- ventilated, temperature-controlled facilities. The correct wattage should be used for a safelight. A filter for the safelight that matches the sensitivity of the film being developed should also be utilized. The light should be positioned at least 4 feet away from the work space. A darkroom light switch should have a delay to minimize any accidental light exposures. Wet and dark areas should be separated to prevent unintended exposures. The images should be processed by technicians wearing appropriate safety equipment. This includes proper gloves and protective eye wear. An eyewash bottle should be kept in the vicinity, in compliance with state, province, and/or federal regulations regarding timely treatment following an accident.

Light leakage is defined as an event which leads to fogging of the images in the radiographs. A check for fogging can be accomplished by placing an open, unprocessed film cassette in the darkroom. Three quarters of the film should be covered with a lightweight paper board for a period of 1 minute. The other portion of the cardboard should be covered for the second minute. The first section should be uncovered during this time. Continue in like manner, until the entire board has had 1 minute of covered exposure. This takes a total of 3 minutes time. On the fourth minute, the film is left uncovered in its entirety so that the film can be totally exposed. After development, any darkened areas on the film will indicate conditions which permit film fogging to occur.

Manual film processing

Processing of film involves the following steps: developing, rinsing (in a stop bath), fixing, washing, and drying. The chemicals must be diluted and mixed according to the manufacturer's directions. The chemical solutions are mixed at a temperature of 20 °C or 68 °F. The manufacturer lists detailed information about the time-temperature development of each chemical. The film should be shaken at regular intervals to prevent any air bubbles from forming while in the developing fluid. The oxidation of developing chemicals can be reduced by keeping lids securely fastened on the tanks. As the developer solution is used, the exposed silver halide crystals are changed to black metallic silver. If the expected density or contrast does not appear, then the solution has weakened and should not be used. The fixer solution is used to remove unexposed, undeveloped silver halide from the image. It also hardens the film. It should be discarded if it takes longer than 2 or 3 minutes for this step to be completed. The process is finished when the image goes from a hazy, cloudy image to a clear image.

Automatic film processing

Mechanized film processors can be employed to provide automated film processing. The film is routed through the chemical solutions and out to a dryer on a roller assembly. The temperature ranges from 20 to 35 °C (77 to 96 °F). Mechanized film processing can take as little as 90 seconds or as long as 8 minutes. The procedures and chemicals are much like those used in the manual processing methods. However, these mechanical chemicals are mixed in a much more concentrated manner. The hardener is mixed directly into the developer solution. There is no rinsing step between the developing and fixing steps in this method. The mechanical process can only be accomplished by maintaining very clean equipment. The rollers, roller racks, and crossover rollers cannot be dirty. Chemicals should be replaced at recommended intervals to give optimum performance in the mechanized film development process.

Radiographic density

Radiographic density ultimately relates to the degree of darkness or blackness present on the developed film's surface. The density level is directly correlated with the number of photons that have affected the film. The density can vary according to the total number of x-rays that come into contact with the intensifying screen, transferring the image to the film. It can also be altered by the penetration strength of the x-rays. Density can be further influenced by the development time and temperature. Focusing filters and grids can make the beam weaker. In addition, tissue density and patient coverings and support pads can lessen the strength of the beam. The beam strength and exposure duration is measured in milliampere-seconds of x-rays that come into contact with the intensifying screen. The more x-rays that come into contact with the intensifying screen (a function of both strength and time), the more densely activated (darkened) is the film. The strength of penetration is determined by the measurement of kVp (kilovoltage peak). The higher kVp settings produce higher energy x-rays. These higher energy x-rays have higher levels of penetration strength. This results in an improved film density. Thicker or denser tissue causes a reduced film density (lighter film). In like manner, thinner tissue causes an increase in film density (darker film).

Radiographic contrast and subject contrast

Black and white can be combined to produce a variety of different shades of gray and degrees of intensity. The degree of difference between the shades is defined as the radiographic contrast. Radiographic contrast can be impacted by the following: kilovoltage, scatter radiation, processing features, and physical aspects. Some examples of physical aspects include beam attenuation and fogging effects. Kilovoltage or kVp has the strongest impact on

- 41 -

radiographic contrast. The x-ray beam is polychromatic, with many wavelengths. Lower kVp ratings offer wider ranges of energy levels. Higher kVp ratings produce more consistent penetration and fewer disparities. Objects along the pathway of the beam scatter the effect. This creates a reduction in the film's contrast and is displayed by overcast shades of gray on the film.

Subject contrast distinguishes between the density and mass of 2 adjacent structures. A high subject contrast will produce a more prominent radiographic contrast. The thickness and density of the anatomic structures being imaged will also impact subject density. Higher tissue density is translated into higher subject density. Bones are an example of an object with high subject density, as bones are more opaque to x-rays, and will thus image as white or light gray on a radiographic image.

Radiation safety

The practice owner should be responsible for applying the appropriate radiological safety procedures in accordance with state or province requirements. These guidelines involve the use of dosimeter devices, efficient radiation detection devices, equipment registration, staff certification, and radiologically appropriate room design. The health department is normally responsible for regulating these devices and safeguards. Trained personnel are necessary to apply the appropriate radiation safety guidelines. Personnel must be able to use the devices correctly, according to instructions received. Every cell in an organism can be affected by ionizing radiation. Ionizing radiation generates charged particles that are able to modify or disintegrate a molecule. Modified molecules may not perform their intended functions appropriately. This can dangerously interrupt the normal functioning of tissues. This harm may not be immediately apparent. Some effects do not become evident for hours, days, months, years, or even generations. Intergenerational delays may occur when damage presents itself only in the genetic makeup of reproductive cells. Other alterations may not be readily apparent because of concurrent tissue restoration. Even so, somatic cell damage may take place throughout the body. The region of the cell most susceptible to the effects of ionizing radiation is the nucleus, and those aspects central to cellular reproduction.

Maximum permissible dose of radiation

Radiation exposure standards are set to ensure patient and staff safety. The maximum radiation exposure allowed is defined in terms of dose rates and exposure time (dose = dose rate x exposure time). Thus, the maximum exposure time permitted is a function of the environmental and occupational dose rate. In clinical settings, the criteria are set according to guidelines issued by the National Committee on Radiation Protection and Measurements (the NCRP). These are derived from the recommendations produced by the International Commission on Radiological Protection (the ICRP).

The NCRP, and almost every province and state, has established radiological protection guidelines. These guidelines specify acceptable rates of exposure when, for example, one is holding an animal for an x-ray (some states, however, prohibit any type of manual animal restraint). To provide an extra measure of protection, staff will wear an individual dosimeter at the work site. It provides a cumulative record of radiation exposure over time, and is evaluated by a federally approved laboratory on a routine basis.

Additional safety practices
Radiation treatments cannot be conducted when a pregnant person is present in the room. When conducting radiological procedures it is best to use nonmanual restraints on the patient, even if the state allows manual restraints, to avoid unnecessary x-ray exposure. Persons in the room should wear the following: protective gloves, thyroid protectors, and aprons. The x-ray machine itself should not be handled without protection. It is necessary to use a 2.5 mm aluminum filter to eradicate the lower-energy portion of the x-ray beam. The x-ray machine requires routine maintenance and calibration. It is important to keep body parts out of the path of the primary beam. This is necessary because of the primary beam's ability to transmit 25% of its radiation through a body shield. The technician should wear a dosimeter next to the outside collar of the apron. Ideally, diagnostic radiographs will be achieved with the fastest (i.e., lowest dosing) film-screen systems employed by the attending technician.

Criteria and principles for positioning and restraint

Non-manual restraint of an animal is always recommended because of its minimization of radiation exposure for staff. Calipers are measuring instruments used to determine the number of centimeters involved in an area to be radiologically exposed. The recommended views are taken from 2 right angles. However, this is not true for thoracic views, contrast studies, equine radiography, and injuries that present only one view option. It is best to achieve a close up shot with the film nearest to the subject as is workable. The beam should be centered over the specified portion of the body. The film is positioned in a parallel direction. The x-ray beam is set perpendicular to the portion of the body to be shot. Some accommodation may be necessary for certain anatomy parts. This accommodation may be in the form of collimating (bringing into a direct line) the machine to use the smallest field available. Extremities are shot with the proximal and distal joints of long bones included in the image. The patient may need to be repositioned to get the best view. It is best to take the time necessary for repositioning so that retakes will not be required.

Contrast media used in contrast radiography

Radiography allows hollow areas of the body (vessels, intestines, etc) to be more meaningfully viewed. Two variations of the contrast medium include positive and negative contrasts. The positive contrast agents are known as radiopaque agents. These agents are found in products like barium and iodine. Radiopaque agents have the capacity to absorb x-rays more thoroughly than the absorption rate found in bones. This causes the structure filled with the radiopaque agent to appear whiter on the film than any other structure in view. Barium is typically employed when examining areas of the gastrointestinal tract. This is an insoluble positive contrast agent. Soluble contrast agents are found in products with iodine. These products are appropriate for the examination of the renal, articular, vascular, myelographic, and gastrointestinal systems. It should be noted that some patients can exhibit toxic reactions to these agents, although these reactions rarely occur. Soluble iodinated contrast agents can be attributed to a hyperosmotic condition.

Negative contrast agents include air and carbon dioxide, and are known as radiolucents. Radiolucent media will show up as black (indicating a void) in radiographs. This is because it is entirely unable to absorb x-rays. Both positive and negative contrast agents are employed by professionals using double-contrast studies.

Sound waves

A wavelength is defined as the span of distance that a wave travels in one repeating cycle. Wavelength is written in an abbreviated international symbolic or notation form as: λ (i.e., the lowercase Greek letter lambda). Audible sound has a wavelength that spans a lengthier distance than the wavelength displayed by an ultrasound. A transducer is a device that converts one form of energy into another form. The defining features of the transducer may influence the wavelength. A second is defined as a unit of time measured in a given cycle. This measurement is applied to number the times a cycle is replicated. The frequency is how many times the cycle occurred. Frequency is given the following symbol: (f). The wavelength will extend for a longer distance or increase as the frequency decreases. The frequency range for ultrasonic waves is measured at 2 to 10 MHz. The frequency range for human auditory perception is approximately 20 Hz–20 khz. Velocity is given the following symbol: (v). Sound velocity is defined as the speed at which a sound wave travels through a medium. The formula for velocity is given as the frequency multiplied by the wavelength.

Transducer

A transducer is a device that transforms one form of energy into another form. The transducer probe is the principal transforming component of the ultrasound machine. This device will transform sound waves into electrical energy, from which an image can be obtained. The sound waves produce echoes that can be received as they bounce back in return. The pulsed-wave transducer is a device that emits a short pulse of sound, and works to send and receive these signals in a patterned sequence. An additional form of a transducer probe is known as a continuous-wave transducer. This device actually utilizes 2 transducers. The first transducer sends out a constant sound wave, while the second transducer continuously receives sound waves as they echo back.

Transducer crystals
Ultrasound devices function with transducer crystals to enhance the electrical energy conversion process. However, a transducer crystal cannot send and receive sound waves simultaneously. Thus, the transducer must perform these functions in an alternating pattern (unless a dual-crystal [continuous] wave transducer is used). Natural crystals are often utilized as transducer crystals. These crystals include: quartz, tourmaline, and Rochelle salts. Some synthetic crystals are also utilized as transducer crystals. Synthetic crystals include the following: lead zirconate titanate, barium titanate, and lithium sulfate. Sound vibrations are promoted via a piezoelectric electric effect. A dampener is applied to terminate the vibrations

after they have been received. Then new echoes received come into contact with the crystals and initiate the vibration again. These vibrating movements back and forth are subsequently transformed into electrical energy.

<u>Linear array transducer</u>
One version of transducer is known as the linear array transducer. The linear array transducer has a tiny row of crystals that operates in a regular rhythm. The linear array transducer produces a composite image from many parallel lines. These lines form an image in a rectangular shape. Thus, the linear array transducer is often best applied to imaging a wide, near field such as transrectals and equine tendons.

<u>Additional types of transducers</u>
Another kind of transducer is known as the mechanical multiple angle or sector scanning transducers. The mechanical sector transducer utilizes one or more crystals in its operations. The device will create an image that has the form of a pie wedge or circle segment. It is often a better choice when deep tissue penetration and a large, far-field view is needed. Another version of a transducer is the phased array sector scanner. This computerized device has the ability to guide ultrasound pulses from about 20 crystals through a particular area. Providing images of time-motion (TM) activity, the phased array sector scanner is best applied to echocardiography. However, this compact device can be an expensive purchase. Another version of a transducer is the broad bandwidth transducer. This version utilizes a piezoelectric ceramic and epoxy material in the probe. It is a lightweight device with a minimum of acoustic impedance. Importantly, these transducers can operate on a variety of frequencies. These frequencies or short-duration pulses are available because of the transducer's ability to transmit over a wide range of bandwidths.

Resolution, lateral resolution, and axial resolution

A properly resolved (clearly seen) image on an ultrasound is defined as 2 small objects in close proximity which can be individually recognized. The frequency of the transducer is critical to the resolution quality of the image. Resolution is increased when higher frequencies are applied. This is due to the shorter wavelength used to gain the image. Lateral resolution refers to the ability to properly resolve 2 objects that are both side-by-side and perpendicular to the beam. The beam functions to visually separate the 2 objects from each other. The degree of lateral resolution is also a function of the beam's width. Objects in parallel position to each other are best able to be identified when they are spaced farther apart than the diameter of the beam. Axial resolution is the ability to resolve 2 objects are located one above another in the beam's pathway. In this situation, greater resolution and differentiation is obtained at lower frequencies.

Sound beam zones

The size and design of the transducer controls the ultrasound beam zones. The near field (also called Fresnel zone) refers to the entire area of the ultrasound beam that precedes the focal point and is most proximal (nearest) the crystal. It is characterized by a narrowing, gradually converging beam shape. The near field is that portion of the ultrasound beam that is closest to the crystal. The narrowest position or spot that is reached is known as the beam's focal point. The shifting of the focal point closer to the image can produce a better resolution of the image. The transducer can be brought into focus by "shaping" (manipulating) the crystal. The focus can also be improved by adding a lens to the transducer. The section of the beam that gets broader, and less intense, as it moves away from the focal point is known as the far field (also called the Fraunhofer zone).

Display formats

The different display formats for ultrasound images include: amplitude mode, brightness mode, and motion mode. The amplitude mode is abbreviated as A-mode. It can provide the depth and dimensions of a target. A-mode is demonstrated as a one-dimensional graph with a succession of rising points. Each rising point stands for a returning echo. A point that is higher on the graph is indicative of a larger, more intense echo coming back. The brightness mode (B-mode) produces a two-dimensional map of data represented by dots or small marks on a graph. The dots represent the returning echo. The deepness of the mirrored image is indicated by the location of the dot on the graph's baseline. The baseline is used to reference the results found.

The motion mode (M-mode) is represented by a one-dimensional wave graph. Its vertical axis indicates the immediate position of the moving reflector. The horizontal axis represents the time. Objects in motion are represented by wavy lines on the graph. Stationary or immobile objects are represented by straight lines on the graph. The M-mode is best applied for cardiac examinations on a patient. The M-mode provides a beneficial evaluation of the condition of cardiac valves, walls, and chamber sizes. These display formats are essential to the ultrasound's ability to provide a display that meets the criterion for each particular purpose sought by the technician obtaining the image.

Attenuation artifacts

Posterior shadowing occurs when an object blocks sound waves from passing deeper into the body. This type of shadowing can be a result of calculi and/or gas in the intestines. Calculi are defined as stones or hard fragments that are formed in the kidney, gallbladder, or urinary bladder. Objects located on the backside of organs filled with fluid may present with enhanced echoes, when compared to adjacent objects or tissues. This enhancement is a result of a fluid's anechoic nature, allowing sound waves to more readily pass through, and thus resulting in acoustic enhancement.

Attenuation artifact occurs when tissues in the near field reduce the intensity of the ultrasound beam, leaving tissues in the focal region and far field poorly imaged. Attenuation artifact may cause a lesion itself to be perceived as a hypoechoic mass or cyst. Hypoechoic conditions exist when certain tissues direct less sound back to the transducer than adjacent tissues. This less reflective tissue creates a darker appearance than the neighboring tissue.

Examples include muscle compared to tendon fiber, soft atherosclerotic plaque, and some tumor tissues.

Doppler imaging

Doppler imaging is beneficial in examining aspects of the body that remain in constant motion. One such part of the body is blood. Doppler imaging uses differences between sound wave frequencies received at a remote point as opposed to the frequency found at the sound's origin to analyze certain characteristics about motion. The difference is most pronounced when there is activity between the original sound and the receiver. Specifically, the sound wave frequency can increase when the receiver is moving towards the originating location of the sound, and it can decrease when the receiver moves away. Thus, the frequency will increase or decrease in relationship to any movement between the receiver and the originating source. The position-dependent wave amplitude changes between a stationary object and one in motion are referred to as a "Doppler shift." In Doppler imaging, a continuous-wave ultrasonic beam is sent to and received back from a part of the body in motion. Using the sound wave frequency data obtained from movement such as blood flow, the blood's velocity can be calculated. Doppler imaging is beneficial in determining whether or not a lesion or a mass exists in a vessel. Doppler imaging can also help in locating portal systemic shunts and in assessing cardiac function and effectiveness in the body, etc.

Sonographic appearance of the heart and spleen

Sonography is an imaging system used to produce a visual likeness of organs found in the body. The heart is visualized using 2 types of sonographic imagery: M-mode or two-dimensional B-mode imaging. Sonograms of the heart require that 2 separate directional views be taken along both the long- and short-axis of the organ. The Doppler imaging technique can then be applied to determine the turbulence and velocity of red blood cells within the heart. For an echocardiogram (cardiac sonogram), the animal should be placed in a lateral recumbent position. The heart is normally ultrasonographically examined by aiming the ultrasound transducer between the fourth and fifth ribs. In this way, it is possible for the transducer beam to reach the heart from the underside of the animal. A hyperechoic appearance is seen in the walls and valves of the heart. A hyperechoic condition results when the tissue or an organ (or parts thereof) are highly reflective of an ultrasound beam, thus producing a brighter or whiter appearance on the ultrasound image than the surrounding tissue.

Sonographic appearance of the liver, gallbladder, and kidneys

The largest part of the spleen is hyperechoic. It has a standard granular profile. It is also surrounded by an illuminated capsule. The patient's spleen should be ultrasonographically imaged from the left side. This side provides the best option for examining the spleen, with the least amount of surrounding tissue interference. The spleen lies just below the skin and facia, behind the stomach and under the diaphragm. Viewing the spleen from the trailing edge of the liver provides important imaging advantages. The liver's outer layer has a thick surface which presents an echogenic disparity that should be avoided. The gallbladder (or cholecyst) is located under the liver. The liver has a multitude of vessels and bile channels. Sonographic images of the gallbladder are displayed as anechoic, as it is largely fluid (bile) filled. Thus, it presents itself as an illuminated wall. Sludge or solid deposits can occasionally be found and visualized in the gallbladder. Animals that have not eaten before a sonogram often have large (i.e., dilated) gallbladder sonographic images. The kidney will present as ovoid or egg-shaped. It will be enclosed by an illuminated capsule, as the cortex of the kidney is hyperechoic. The medulla of the kidney presents itself as anechoic. The pelvic fat will be displayed as an illuminated central zone. The sagittal view should be measured to determine the size.

Sonographic appearance of the bladder, prostate, and uterus

A sonographic image of the urinary bladder is typically dark, as it is fluid filled and thus is relatively anechoic. However, the bladder has a wall that presents itself as hyperechoic, and it is not unusual to find debris in the bladder that aids in visualization. In the male, the prostate can be ultrasonographically located by following the urethra to the pelvic inlet. The urethra is encircled by the prostate. The prostate is composed of 2 lobes. The prostate has an illuminated capsule in its ultrasonographic image. In the female, the uterus is evident as the organ adjacent to an enlarged bladder. The wall of the uterus is hypoechoic. The optimum time to discover an early uterine pregnancy in small animals is at about 30 days into gestation. In horses, the optimum early confirmation time is around 11-14 days into the gestation period. At these junctures, the sonographic equipment should be able to detect viable embryos in their gestational sacs. However, it can often be hard to distinguish the exact number of fetuses inside the sac. This is due to the problem of superimposition and the usual presence of gas in the intestines.

Sonographic appearance of the stomach, bowel, pancreas, and adrenal gland

The presence of gas or flatus in the abdomen and intestines presents a routine obstacle in ultrasonography. This is because air is hyperechoic and thus intestinal flatus limits the imaging of anything in the far field behind it. Even so, the intestinal walls on a sonographic image will look white or dark gray on the screen. Depending upon its contents, the stomach may be hypoechoic. However, the rugal folds of the stomach are usually visible in the image created. The pancreas is sandwiched between the spleen and the stomach. It is adjacent to the duodenum. The pancreas is a digestive and endocrine gland found in the body. The adrenal gland appears as a standard (isoechoic) gray color. The adrenal gland is responsible for the secretion of hormones in the body. The adrenal gland itself is hypoechoic. As reference points, the cranial pole of the kidney is situated toward the middle of the adrenal gland. The renal artery is next to the caudal pole found in the adrenal gland. The renal artery connects to the aorta.

Imaging techniques

Computerized axial tomography
Computerized axial tomography (i.e., a "CAT" scan) is primarily employed as a diagnostic test to determine the health of the central and peripheral nervous system, although it is also used for many other kinds of evaluations. This imaging technique can detect numerous forms of disease in a variety of animals. However, it is also one of the costliest examinations used by veterinarians. The animal having this procedure will require general anesthesia to limit movement. The equipment used in computerized tomography requires that the patient be moved slowly through a circular gantry while remaining virtually motionless. This circular segment of the machine holds the x-ray tube and detectors. The equipment has the capability of moving completely around the patient, encompassing 360 degrees in total. Each movement of the scanner produces a recording of a single cross-sectional slice of data. This recording is created when x-rays are picked up by the scanner. The x-rays are transformed into electronic signals with a wide range of intensity levels. These varying levels are produced through radiant attenuation. The image is then computed and shown in a re-creation produced by the computer.

Nuclear scintigraphy
In nuclear scintigraphy imaging, the patient can be given gamma emissions from radioactive material or radionuclides applied by a variety of methods. These methods include intravenous injections, transcolonic applications, or aerosol insufflation (i.e., blown into or onto the body). The radioactive material is picked up by sensors found in the gamma scintillation camera. The organ is then pictured on x-ray film, formatted in black and white shades of varying contrast.

Clinical nuclear scintigraphy is typically performed on the thyroid, bone, and liver. The results derived from this technique provide physiological, pharmacological, and kinetic data. Nuclear scintigraphy is beneficial in many treatments provided to horses. However, the handler and persons coming into contact with the horse having this procedure should use the recommended safety equipment. This equipment should prevent undue exposure to the harmful effects of radioactive material. The animal will expel the radiopharmaceutical elements in its bodily waste. The contaminated urine and feces is normally expelled within 24 to 72 hours after the procedure was completed.

Magnetic resonance imaging
Magnetic resonance imaging (MRI) produces cross-sectional images of anatomy. This technique has some shared characteristics with those found in computerized axial tomography. However, magnetic resonance imaging does not employ the use of ionizing radiation to create a likeness of the tissues or organs. Instead, it incorporates a magnetic field to produce the desired image being scanned. Enclosed coils in the device are able to transmit and receive magnetic field signals. Then the computer organizes those signals into an image. Magnetic resonance imaging provides an image resolution that has a better quality than other techniques used. Indeed, this device is sensitive enough to display detailed portions of an

animal's anatomy and tissue makeup. Magnetic resonance imaging particularly lends itself to head and spine appraisals that require more intricate images to be produced.

Important terms

Amplitude: The intensity or height of a wave.

Time period: The equivalent of one cycle of the wave. This is given the symbol (T).

Attenuation: A loss of vitality, amplitude, or power. With sound, this occurs when intensity is lost as an ultrasound beam passes through tissue. The loss can be attributed to the way the beam is absorbed into the tissue as it makes its way through. The absorption process creates heat and results in a loss of energy. Tissue that has sound refractory characteristics can scatter the sound in a multitude of directions.

Acoustic impedance: The capability of something to withstand or resist sound conduction. The density of tissue may be reflected in its degree of impedance. However, both air (not dense) and bone (very dense) will significantly obstruct the passage of sound. Thus, both bone and air have a high rate of acoustic impedance, despite their widely differing density. On the whole, however, tissues respond favorably to the passage of sound waves. Therefore, most bodily tissues have a low rate of acoustic impedance.

Echogenic: Tissues with the capacity to produce return echoes. These echoes are singled out by the transducer, and displayed in a black and white image (with varying gray tones) that represents these tissues. Organs in proximity to each other will produce a larger echo reflection, indicating the gap between each organ.

Sonolucent (also called echolucent): Something that does not reflect sound, and thus produces no echo.

Anechoic: An absence of echoes. A condition sometimes characteristic of chambers, spaces, or fluid-filled areas, where the sounds pass deeper into the tissue without producing returning echoes from that area. This produces a black image on the viewing screen, which sometimes represents tissue saturated with fluid.

Hyperechoic: Strong echo reflection. Also, a greater amplitude wave return. The result is a whiter image appearance from the high degree of sound that is transmitted back to the transducer. Examples of hyperechoic tissues include bone, tendons, and ligaments when perpendicular to the beam.

Hypocholic: Giving back few echoes. A condition where less sound echoes back to the transducer, as compared with adjacent tissue. This less reflective tissue creates a darker ultrasound image. Examples include: muscle as compared to tendon fiber, soft atherosclerotic plaque, and some tumor tissue.

Isoechoic: Similar amplitude wave returns. Areas of similar echogenicity are considered to be isoechoic to each other.

Propagation artifacts: Reverberations, refraction, and mirror images. Reverberations are exhibited as linear echoes. Reverberations are a result of sounds reflected between a strong reflector and the transducer in a continuous pattern. An example of a strong reflective (i.e., reverberation-prone) surface is illustrated by bones. Refractions are a result of sound beams changing directions as they are bounced off one medium and strike another medium's surface. Refractions are to blame for the manifestation of organs in unusual positions. An example of this is when an image is duplicated and appears as if it exists on both sides of a reflecting axis.

This phenomenon is often due to the close proximity of strongly reflective organ to the reflector. This is a typical occurrence in ultrasound images taken of the liver and of the diaphragm.

Attenuation artifacts: Include acoustic shadowing and acoustic enhancement. Acoustic shadowing is found when an object reflects a sound wave in its entirety, producing an acoustic shadow of the actual structure. Acoustic enhancement occurs when a propagated wave passes largely unimpeded through an anechoic structure, resulting in an artificially strong wave and echo from otherwise deeper tissues.

Anesthesia and Analgesia

Analgesic/anti-inflammatory drugs

Opioid or narcotic analgesics, corticosteroids, and nonsteroidal anti-inflammatory drugs are defined as analgesic and/or anti-inflammatory drugs. The function of these drugs is to provide immediate pain relief and ongoing control. Nonsteroidal anti-inflammatory drugs may also be referred to by their acronym "NSAIDs." Common NSAIDs include phenylbutazone, aspirin, ibuprofen, etodolac, and carprofen. Nearly all NSAIDs work to block the prostaglandin production that results from the inflammatory process. However, NSAIDs are not useful in counteracting visceral (organ) pain nor the pain associated with broken bones, as they do not produce sufficient analgesic effects. By contrast, opioid analgesics can entirely block all awareness of neural pain impulses. Thus, opioids can control more intense pain symptoms, such as those related to visceral pain and the pain of broken bones. Morphine, meperidine, oxymorphone, butorphanol, and codeine are all types of opioid pain control medications. Many of the perianesthetic medications are also opioids. These medications work as both analgesics and sedatives. Many sedatives can also be effective as tranquilizers. Corticosteroids are anti-inflammatory drugs which can also relieve pain. However, it is important to use caution with these drugs, as they can have negative effects on the endocrine and immune systems. The most widely used corticosteroids are dexamethasone and prednisone.

General anesthesia and euthanizing

General anesthesia serves to bring a patient into a coma-like state of deep unconsciousness, sufficient to produce a loss of all sensation. General anesthetics are administered to the patient as inhalants or injectables. Death can occur if an overdose of some general anesthetics occurs.

Nearly all animal euthanizing agents utilize sodium pentobarbital as the primary active agent. Pentobarbital, without any other additives, is rated as a Schedule II (C-II) drug by the DEA. However, some pentobarbital-based euthanizing agents have additives that work as cardiac depressives. These combined drugs are then reclassified as C-III. Pentobarbital-based animal euthanasia drugs with cardiac depressive additives include Euthanasia-D with phenytoin, and FP-3 (Vortech) with lidocaine.

Sodium pentobarbital injected perivascularly has the ability to induce necrosis. Necrosis is described as the death and decay of tissues or organs within the body. Conversely, lower-dose sodium pentobarbital also has the ability to postpone or prevent death in some cases. Animals that will be consumed as food must not receive any general anesthetics due to the danger that residual medications can be passed on to the human consumer.

Preanesthetic medication

Pre-anesthetic medication lowers the stress level of an animal, when it is given before a procedure. This medication produces a state that supports a smooth induction and effective recovery period. The patient that receives a preanesthetic may well benefit from a reduced need for anesthesia induction and maintenance medications. Preanesthetic medication may also produce some intraoperative and postoperative analgesic effects. These medications have also been known to lower certain secretion levels and to reduce certain autonomic reflexes. This effect gives the handler a more manageable animal that is easier and safer to handle.

Pre-anesthetic medication can remain effective for a period of up to 2 hours, and can be given to the patient by a variety of means. The most common administration is through an intramuscular (or IM) injection. An intravenous (or IV) injection works faster than other methods. However, an IV injection should be given with careful consideration, as administration via this route may induce certain temporary behavior and personality changes. Various side effects from preanesthetic drugs are associated with xylazine, acepromazine, opioids, and diazepam. Additionally, the application of preanesthetic medication can come with some drawbacks. Specifically, time and medication cost factors are involved. However, some of these costs can be counterbalanced though the reduced need for subsequent induction and maintenance agents. Most preanesthetic medications will reach maximum effectiveness levels approximately 20 minutes after an intramuscular injection.

Anticholinergics

Anticholinergic medications may be used to block nerve impulses from reaching the vagus nerve. Examples of anticholinergics include atropine and glycopyrrolate. Pharmacologically blocking this nerve with a vagolytic medication is necessary when the veterinarian is treating bradycardia in a patient. Anticholinergics and opioids can be used in conjunction with each other. The synergistic effects of these drugs can produce lower levels of salivary and tear secretions. Anticholinergics can also diminish bronchodilation. Contraindications associated with anticholinergics include administration to patients at high risk for tachycardia (often geriatric patients), those with a history of congestive heart failure, and patients with constipation or ileus.

Phenothiazines

Occasionally, healthy animals will be scheduled for an elective surgery. These animals can be given phenothiazine, which provides a sedation effect. Phenothiazines include acepromazine and chlorpromazine. Phenothiazines are also given to patients in need of an antiemetic to stop nausea and vomiting. Acepromazine is contraindicated for any patient with a history of convulsions, epilepsy, or head injuries. Acepromazine is known to decrease the threshold level for seizure activity. Phenothiazine-induced peripheral vasodilation in patients with symptoms of shock or hypothermia may cause hypotension (i.e., low blood pressure). Patients with depression or liver or kidney diseases should not be prescribed phenothiazines.

- 53 -

These drugs should only be given to the very young or old with careful observation. A lower dose or alternate medications such as benzodiazepines may be given instead.

Unexpected antihistamine effects can occur when animals are not given a medication-specific allergy test beforehand. Some animals experience adverse effects from taking phenothiazines. These effects include abnormal heartbeat, an unexpected reaction of excitability replacing the desired effect of sedation, and personality changes. These side effects normally subside within 48 hours of taking the medication.

Benzodiazepines

Patients that have epileptic fits or convulsions may find treatment with benzodiazepines beneficial. Others who may benefit are patients that require emotionally traumatic cerebrospinal fluid tap or myelograms. Benzodiazepines are used as tranquilizers. Drugs containing benzodiazepines include the following: diazepam or Valium, zolazepam, midazolam or Versed, and lorazepam or Ativan. All of these variations of the drug may result in depression of the cardiovascular or respiratory systems. However, the remote risk has been determined to be acceptable for both geriatric and pediatric patients. Candidates found to derive the greatest benefits from the drug are elderly, depressed, and/or nervous patients. Benzodiazepines used in conjunction with ketamine may serve as an effective general anesthetic induction agent.

Diazepam is soluble when placed in oil. However, water does not dissolve diazepam. Diazepam may work faster when it is used in conjunction with other drugs. Opioids like butorphanol and oxymorphone easily mix with the midazolam. Midazolam is a medication that is known to be water-soluble.

α2-agonists

Medications that are α2-agonists (alpha-2 agonists) provide sedation, analgesia, muscle relaxation, and anxiolysis. Some α2-agonists include xylazine, romifidine, detomidine, and medetomidine. Xylazine is also known as Rompun and Anased. Detomidine is also known as Dormosedan. Medetomidine is also known as Domitor. α2-agonists are not to be used as preanesthetic medications. Instead, this medication is more suitable for general sedation purposes. The potential for side effects exceeds its benefits as a preanesthetic medication. A vicious animal destined to be euthanized can be given α2-agonists to produce a sedative effect. This medication is also beneficial when given as an analgesic or pain reliever. However, the relief will only last for about 16 to 20 minutes. There is a 50% chance that dogs will become nauseated to the point of vomiting when given this drug. This chance increases to 90% when the medication is given to cats. There are 2 α2-agonists employed for treatments in horses. These are xylazine and detomidine. Ruminants may be given a significantly lower dose of xylazine.

Ignoring the contraindications associated with α2-agonists can produce serious risks for a patient. These risks include cardiac disease, respiratory disease, and liver or kidney disease.

Dogs in a state of shock should not be given this medication. In addition, dogs in a state of incapacitation should not be treated with this class of drug. Other concurrent conditions such as extreme heat or fatigue can produce stress in the animal that can be harmful in conjunction with this medication. Intravenous administration of this medication may produce serious side effects. The animal may experience temporary behavioral and personality changes. Patients given this medication when suffering from dehydration may suffer from reduced pancreatic secretions, resulting in transient hyperglycemia. Opioids may exaggerate these side effects. The effects of xylazine can be reversed by Yohimbine or tolazoline. Another name for Yohimbine is Yobine. Atipamezole is a reversal agent used to counteract medetomidine. Another name for Atipamezole is Antisedan.

Opioids

The following medications are opioids: morphine, oxymorphone or Numorphan, butorphanol or Torbugesic and Torbutrol, hydromorphone, meperidine or Demerol, Pethidine, and fentanyl. Opioids have the following effects on the body: analgesia, sedation, dysphoria, euphoria, and excitability. These effects are precipitated by the drug's interaction between one or more dedicated receptors in the brain and spinal cord in various reversible combinations. Opioids can act as an agonist or antagonist against each dedicated receptor. Preanalgesia medication is given to the patient as an induction agent or for a more balanced anesthesia transition. It also aids in controlling pain after the surgery. The effects of this medication can be reversed by giving the patient a pure antagonist agent. Opioids are categorized as narcotics in Canada and as Schedule II drugs in the United States. Neither country allows the dispensing of these medications without a prescription from a licensed physician or veterinarian.

Phencyclidines

Phencyclidines are available under the following names: Ketamine or Ketaset, Ketalean, Vetalar, and tiletamine hydrochloride. Tiletamine hydrochloride is a combination of zolazepam and Telazol. Another name for phencyclidines is cycloheximide. Patients that need to remain immobile will benefit from the application of this drug in their treatment. This drug is a beneficial preanesthetic when applied to the mucous membranes in the mouth or oral cavity. Felines are the only animals that can take phencyclidines as a solitary form of medication. Other animals should never have this medication in solitary form. Dogs do not respond well to phencyclidine as a preanesthetic medication. It is best to avoid its use in patients with a history of seizure activity. It is best to avoid use for patients with suspected brain herniation or suspected perforation of the eye chamber. Visceral analgesia (pain relief for pain arising in the internal organs) is inadequate. However, the response is much better when given for the purpose of peripheral analgesia. It should be noted that the animal's recovery period after being given this drug may be extensive and unpredictable.

Neuroleptanalgesics and barbiturates

Neuroleptanalgesics are combinations of analgesics with a neuroleptic tranquilizer. Versions of this drug include oxymorphone and acepromazine. Neuroleptanalgesics are employed when it is necessary to produce a deep sedative effect. The dose can be reduced for less extensive procedures, resulting in shorter durations. These shorter time frames may include treatments involving the suturing of an injury or the removal of porcupine quills. Neuroleptanalgesics are beneficial in the treatment of patients with conditions resulting in cardiac distress or shock. Naloxone or nalbuphine are reversal agents for neuroleptanalgesics. Some side effects include hyperactivity, auditory stimuli, defecating, vomiting, panting, and in some cases, bradycardia.

Barbiturates can be used for sedation, as anticonvulsants, and for general anesthesia. This drug can serve as an induction agent prior to endotracheal intubation. The drug may be given as an inhalant anesthetic for maintenance purposes. In some cases the drug will produce unconsciousness in the patient. Two common barbiturates are phenobarbital and pentobarbital. Barbiturates are considered sedative-hypnotic medications. This category of drugs can also be applied to depress respiration and the cardiovascular system in general. The effects of barbiturates are not reversible and no other medication can fully counterbalance their effects. Barbiturates bind to proteins in the body. Thus, the rate and amount of absorption can change when the level of plasma protein is altered.

The most widespread use of phenobarbital in veterinarian medicine is as a sedative for dogs. This drug can be used to calm animals that have reached a level of high excitement. It is also beneficial when used as an anticonvulsant. Varying the dosage may cause the drug to last for shorter or longer periods of time. When given in a high dose, it may have sedative effects for a period ranging up to 24 hours. Phenobarbital is also used for seizure control. Sedation is achieved when the drug is given to the patient by intramuscular means. It has no negative effects upon tissue. The drug will reach its optimum effect about 5 minutes following the injection. Intravenous administration works more quickly, and the patient may respond after only 1 minute following administration. The patient should exhibit a strong effect from the medication. Sheep take longer to recover from this medication than any other type of animal. The majority of animal species will respond quickly and have an easier recovery period when given this drug.

Pentobarbital has been replaced with ultra-short acting barbiturates. In the past it was often employed for the purpose of anesthesia inductions. Pentobarbital may also be given with phenobarbital. While it is not an anticonvulsant, its sedative properties can reduce symptoms while waiting for the phenobarbital to take effect.

Propofol

Propofol is also known as Diprivan or Rapinovet. This drug is useful in veterinary medicine for the following purposes: sedation, anesthesia induction, and anesthesia maintenance. It is also effective as an anticonvulsant. Propofol usually results in an induction procedure that is

- 56 -

relatively easy and stress free. The drug known as propofol is a short-acting sedative that is rapidly dispersed throughout the body, including the brain. Although it is oil-soluble, the medication is not retained in the muscle or fat and is metabolized out of the body very quickly by the liver. Metabolic clearance of this drug is faster than required for barbiturates. This is also the preferred preanesthetic induction medication for the sight hound breeds (i.e., whippets, greyhounds, Deerhounds, Irish Wolfhounds, Pharaoh Hounds, Afghan Hounds, Salukis, Borzois, Ibizan Hounds, Basenjis, Rhodesian Ridgebacks, and a select few others). It is also preferred for low body mass index (skinny) patients. Further, it is useful as an injectable maintenance anesthesia due to its fast-acting properties. It should be noted that propofol may cause tachycardia, bradycardia, temporary arterial and venous dilation, and depressed cardiac contractility. Typically, however, this medication has no effect on the cardiovascular system.

Etomidate

Etomidate is also known by the name Amidate. This drug is used as an anesthesia induction agent. It is considered to be safe and fast acting. It is dispersed rapidly throughout the body and does not build up in any tissues or organs. An animal is administered the drug through a repeated bolus or continuous infusion. During this time the animal may suffer from vomiting, diarrhea, and excitement. This can be attributed to the drug, the induction process, and/or postanesthesia effects. The animal may show brief signs of apnea (a pause in breathing), and thus should be monitored carefully.

Etomidate is a medication that can cross the placental barrier. However, it is usually harmless due to the liver's ability to metabolize the drug quickly. Etomidate is able to mildly depress the respiratory system. It can also have a rare side effect that results in extreme muscle rigidity and seizures in horses and cattle. An animal may experience a great deal of pain when given an IV injection of etomidate. Thus, some veterinarians also administer lidocaine for pain control. The injection can also result in phlebitis or inflammation of the veins. However, inflammation more often occurs in smaller-sized veins.

Guaifenesin and fentanyl

Guaifenesin is also known as glycerol guaiacolate. This drug is described as a decongestant and antitussive. Guaifenesin works on the central nervous system and skeletal muscles as a relaxant. It is most often used for treatment in large animals. This medication can serve well for anesthesia induction and recovery. The animal will experience only mild effects on the respiratory and cardiac systems. While the drug is able to cross the placental barrier, the fetus should not experience any harmful effects. Fentanyl is most often used as an analgesic (pain reliever). Unconsciousness can result from the use of fentanyl. Mainly, this drug is employed in conjunction with a tranquilizer, sedative, or benzodiazepine. It is considered to be an injectable induction agent. This drug does not cause problems with apnea. While it can cause contractility or cardiac output changes, it is not contraindicated for most high-risk patients. Fentanyl is usually classified as a neuroleptanalgesic.

Inhalation anesthesia

There are certain factors that should be recognized when using inhalation anesthetic medications. First, the lungs absorb inhalation anesthesia as either gases or vapors. The medication is rapidly carried from the alveoli or air sacs in the lungs to the brain and body. During initial dispersal, this medication remains in the same chemical form (it has not yet been changed by the liver or other metabolic events). The amount ultimately delivered to the patient can be impacted by variables such as vapor pressure, boiling point, and the anesthetic delivery system used. The medication has to be carried through the lungs subject to alveolar partial pressure, the inspired concentration, and the alveolar concentration. To be effective, the tissues must be able to readily absorb the medication. Delivery from the lungs to the brain is contingent upon the drug's solubility, the relative rate of blood flow in the arteries and tissues, the strength of the anesthetic, the tissue type, and the blood saturation of the tissues. MAC is the acronym for minimal alveolar concentration. This abbreviation stands for the level of anesthetic vapor concentration in the lungs needed to prevent a motor response to surgical pain in 50% of all patients. The potency level rises as the MAC number is reduced.

Inhalation anesthesia has certain advantages over injectable medications. These advantages include the anesthetic depths achieved and the ease in regulation. The patient's recovery is also considered to be more rapid. Further, inhalation anesthesia provides a drug that is metabolized at a nominal rate. This is a result of the body's ability to easily expel the excess medication through the respiration process.

A patient's airway is used when an endotracheal tube is applied. The patient will require assisted breathing at this juncture. Inhalation anesthesia should be delivered in an initial dose that is considered a fully safe concentration, and then increased as needed. This will allow the induction of anesthesia without undue depression of the respiratory and cardiovascular systems. Inhalation anesthesia typically has both analgesic and muscle relaxant properties, and both will benefit the patient. Patient recovery is considered to be more rapid due to the capacity of these medications to be quickly eliminated from the body. Inhalation medications do not persist or accumulate within the body's tissues or systems.

Halothane

One of the benefits of halothane involves its modest respiratory depression effects. Further, it is not considered to be nephrotoxic, and can be mask induced. Some drawbacks of halothane anesthesia are found in the risk to the patient of cardiac arrhythmias, hypotension from cardiac depression, minimal analgesic or pain-relieving impact, and hepatotoxic effects. The patient should be given an out-of-circle precision vaporizer to maintain the required elevated vapor pressure. This practice provides the patient with the safest exposure to Halothane. Methoxyflurane has a lower solubility factor than halothane. This creates a faster rate of anesthesia induction and recovery level for the patient. The veterinarian can thus respond to adjustments needed in the concentration levels at a faster pace. MAC is the acronym for minimal alveolar concentration. The MAC of halothane is 0.8%. This refers to the level of anesthetic vapor concentration in the lungs needed to prevent a motor response to surgical pain in 50% of all patients. The potency level rises when the MAC is reduced.

Isoflurane

Isoflurane is known to induce only insignificant metabolic changes in the liver. Isoflurane is also considered to be a prudent treatment as related to the cardiovascular system. Indeed, this drug exhibits low arrhythmogenicity even while simultaneously enhancing cardiac productivity. Isoflurane is a medication that rapidly induces anesthesia, and with a shorter recovery period than many other medications. The dosage of this drug can be also be adjusted easily, given the drug's low solubility characteristics. In fact, it offers a much quicker dosage adjustment and response time than that available through the drug halothane. Even so, there are some problems associated with isoflurane. These issues pertain to respiratory depression, difficult recovery periods, and rising costs, as both halothane and isoflurane require an out-of-circle precision vaporizer to raise vapor pressures. Isoflurane produces blood pressures associated with normal rates when linked with vasodilation. The MAC of isoflurane for canines is 1.2%. The MAC of isoflurane in cats is at 1.6%. This refers to the level of anesthetic vapor concentration in the lungs needed to prevent a motor response to surgical pain in 50% of all patients. The potency level rises when the MAC is reduced.

Sevoflurane

Sevoflurane is considered to have a very low solubility, and therefore provides speedy anesthesia induction and recovery periods. Further, it does not readily induce cardiac arrhythmias. The animal should also respond with a superior rate of muscle relaxation. The drug has an analgesic quality used to bring pain relief to the patient. Sevoflurane is considered to be a particularly appropriate analgesic inhalant for the majority of avian or bird species. Sevoflurane is considered to be less overpowering than other inhalants. Thus, it leaves the patient with no symptoms resembling a hangover, as might otherwise be expected from the use of a psychoactive drug. Sevoflurane and isoflurane both produce respiratory depression in the patient. Sevoflurane can also cross the placental barrier. This can result in concurrent fetal depression. Finally, this drug is typically more costly than either halothane or isoflurane. Sevoflurane is MAC rated at 2.4%. MAC is the acronym for minimal alveolar concentration. This refers to the level of anesthetic vapor concentration in the lungs needed to prevent a motor response to surgical pain in 50% of all patients. The potency level rises when the MAC number is reduced.

Desflurane

The MAC rating for Desflurane is 7.2%. This refers to the level Desflurane promotes rapid anesthesia induction and recovery. This can be attributed to the drug's low solubility and consequent rapid dispersion. It does not display a tendency for either hepatotoxicity or nephrotoxicity. Desflurane requires the use of a unique, electrically heated vaporizer in its administration. This type of vaporizer can be extremely costly to purchase. Further, Desflurane has a pungent odor that can irritate the respiratory tract. Thus, patients tend to cough and hold their breath when being administered this drug. Some animal species will experience a malignant hyperthermia from the use of this drug. Other patients may recover before treatment is finished. Patients that experience a premature recovery will need more sedation given immediately.

Nitrous oxide

Nitrous oxide (chemical symbol: N_2O) is a very weak general anesthetic with a MAC rating of 105%. However, it is very effective as a "carrier gas" for other more powerful anesthetics. Mixed in a 2:1 ratio with oxygen, it serves to increase the rate of inhalation induction in the patient. At the start of anesthesia induction, large quantities of nitrous oxide are distributed from the alveoli into the bloodstream. For some animals (depending upon the procedure), N_2O alone may provide sufficient anesthesia. Other animals may require further analgesics to be administered. Nitrous oxide has an immediate effect due to the body's inability to metabolize the medication (less than 0.004% of this gas is metabolized). The body's cardiovascular and respiratory system suffers little effect from the application of this medication. With a MAC rating over 100%, another medication must be used in conjunction with N_2O if general anesthesia is required. Further, the inspiration levels of O_2 drop to 33% when N_2O is administered. This drop in levels can endanger the patient. The patient may suffer from of hypoxia if there is a history of respiratory problems. Further, N_2O is contraindicated in animals with gas-occupying conditions such as gastric dilation, intestinal obstruction, or pneumothorax.

Anesthesia machine

An anesthesia machine is fashioned from the following: medical gas cylinders, a regulator, flowmeter, vaporizer, inhalation or exhalation flutter valves, check valves, y-connector, a rebreathing bag or reservoir bag, carbon dioxide absorber, soda lime canister, exhaust valve, manometer, oxygen flush valve, scavenger system, and a negative pressure relief valve. The gas cylinders hold compressed gas which is subjected to extreme pressures. Full containers of oxygen are pressurized at around 2000-2200 psi. (pounds per square inch). Full containers of nitrous oxide are pressurized from 750-770 psi. A regulator can reduce the pressure of the gas exiting to around 50 psi. The flowmeter sets the gas delivery at a certain rate. The flowmeter can further reduce the pressure to approximately 15 psi. The liquid anesthetic is changed to a vapor with the vaporizer. It regulates the quantity of anesthesia combined with the carrier gas. The circle system utilizes a check valve to ensure and control the unidirectional flow of gas. The parts of an anesthesia machine and describe functions of the check valves, y-connector, reservoir bag, carbon dioxide absorber, exhaust valve, manometer, oxygen flush valve, scavenger system, and the negative pressure relief valve.

The circle system's inspiration and expiration tubes are linked to the endotracheal tube with a y-connector. The reservoir bag achieves an improved form of breathing with its gas reservoir. Animal size is a crucial variable that must be accounted for in the gas flow rate. Thus, minimum gas volume requirements are around 60 mL/kg of patient weight. The circle system's carbon dioxide absorber removes the carbon dioxide from the expired gas. The tanks must be replaced every 6 to 8 hours when in use. The exhaust valve is utilized in extracting the exhaust gas from the machine into the scavenger system. The manometer can detect the amount of pressure of gas in the lungs and airway of the patient. It measures the pressure using the following increments: mm of Hg or cm of H2O. The system can be cleansed with pure oxygen by releasing the oxygen flush valve. The waste gas is accumulated and directed out of the building. A second alternative allows the waste anesthesia to be extracted by a charcoal canister in the scavenger system. The negative relief valve is described as a safety valve that releases to allow room air in when a negative pressure is formed.

Maintenance

The oxygen tanks should be turned off when not in use. This reduces any additional pressure on the oxygen tank regulator. Removable parts of the anesthesia machine can be cleaned with a gentle soapy solution. Any parts that have come into contact with the patient should be cleansed. Removable parts should be placed in a tub of cold disinfectant solution to soak. Following the soak, the parts should be thoroughly rinsed and left to air dry. Cleaning should be performed following each anesthesia induction. Vaporizers should be turned off when not in use. In addition, these appliances should be emptied to prevent any undue buildup of preservatives or residue. A good rule is to check the color of the barium hydroxide or soda lime granules. A color change is a good indication that it is time to change the solution. If the substance becomes rigid and/or brittle, then it should be replaced. It is important to note that rubber does require replacing, as it wears out with use.

Closed rebreathing systems

Rebreathing or circle systems operate by circulating a combination of expired and fresh gases. The amount of CO2 in the inhaled gas is regulated by the flow rate of the fresh air and the presence or absence of a CO2 absorber. The fresh gas flow rate should not exceed the metabolic oxygen expenditure of the patient. This rate is typically 5 to 10 mL/kg/minute with a closed rebreathing system. The pop-off valve can be in the closed position during operation of the system. Incoming fresh gases are recirculated in combination with expired gases that have gone through a CO2 extraction process. If the CO2 absorber is not working effectively, then the patient can be exposed to unhealthy levels of CO2. It is important to consistently monitor the operation to keep the O2 flow at the desired metabolic levels. This monitoring will prevent undue pressure from developing in the rebreathing system's operation.

Universal F-circuit

A modified circle system contains a universal F-circuit with the inspiration hose on the inside of the expiration hose. This system requires the following: a CO2 absorber, rebreathing bag, unidirectional valves, pop-off valve, and a scavenger. The expired gases heat the inward-bound fresh gases. The universal F-circuit is lightweight. It is less cumbersome than the circle system version. It also incorporates safety measures through an end-of-the-inspiration hose and end-of-the-expiration hose pull away connection. This juncture disconnects when the circuit is stretched. The empty space of this system is fashioned like the one found in the circle system. However, the empty space does increase when the hoses stretch.

Bain system

The Bain system is also known as the Bain coaxial anesthesia circuit. It holds a tube inside another tube. The interior tube allows fresh gas to flow in, and the exterior tube conducts exhaled gasses away. The Bain system does not incorporate a CO_2 absorber. Instead, it incorporates a rebreathing bag sandwiched between the reservoir bag and scavenger. The following is drawn from the interior tube during the patient's inspiration or inhalation process: fresh gases, either 100% fresh gas or a mixture of fresh and expired gases. A nonrebreathing system utilizes the fresh flow rate of 200 to 300 mL/kg/minute in the mechanism. A partial breathing system can utilize a flow rate of 130 to 200 mL/kg/minute in the system. The Bain system is compact and light. It has a minimum amount of empty space, which promotes effortless breathing. This is an ideal system for a patient that is under 7 kg or 15 lb. The Bain system is also ideal for treatments that are applied to the head or where there is a need for a great deal of physical manipulation of the patient during a procedure.

Precision and nonprecision vaporizers

A precision vaporizer incorporates an anesthetic vapor concentration that is regulated independently, and based on the time, temperature, and fresh gas flow rate. An anesthetist can compensate for the temperature flow rate manually. This can be accomplished with a vaporizer. The percentage of the anesthetic is fixed according to dials, charts, and/or mathematical calculations. It is impossible for the patient to physically extract gases out of a precision vaporizer. This is due to the internal resistance inherent in the device. The problem is alleviated with an out-of-circle position. The complexity of this device requires particular skill when it is being serviced. Nonprecision vaporizers are not appropriate for the administration of a specific, continuous percentage of anesthesia. This is because nonprecision vaporizers are unable to accommodate the following variables: changes in temperature, fresh gas flow rates, ventilation changes, liquid and wick surfaces, and the volume of liquid anesthetic. Thus, these vaporizers do not lend to an accurate calculation and consistent maintenance of the percentage of anesthetic given to the patient. Even so, the low internal resistance allows an in-the-circle application, and this application can include an out-of-circle operation. The nonlinear concentrations given make it hard to regulate the anesthesia depth. However, this simple device does not require as much maintenance as the precision vaporizer requires.

Eye position and palpebral reflex

Patients that are in stage III, plane 2 of anesthesia will not exhibit eyeball movement, and the pupils will begin to dilate and the eye will rotate to a ventral medial (central) position. In dogs and cats, the eyeball rotates down when under halothane, isoflurane, barbiturate, and propofol anesthesia, and does not revert to a central position until deeper in plane 3. Patients that exhibit any eye movement or blinking are not sedated heavily enough for surgery to commence. The veterinarian can gently touch the medial or lateral canthus of the eyelid to stimulate the palpebral (i.e., pertaining to the eyelid) reflex or blinking reflex in the eyes. The patient's medial palpebral reflex will fade away after the lateral reflex becomes more intense. In stage III, plane 2 of anesthesia the medication causes the patient's reflex to grow slower and weaker until it ebbs to nothing. The only acceptable reflex is found in that of a mild medial palpebral reflex that can be viewed after an analgesic has been given to the patient. This reflex is also present when an injectable anesthesia is used as a solitary medication. It may also be present when methoxyflurane is used. The corneal reflex disappears at the deeper end of plane 2. Gentle palpation of the lateral aspect of the cornea will produce eyelid closure if the reflex is still intact. If not, sedation may need to be lightened. This reflex is more difficult to determine if the eyeball is significantly rotated downward, as occurs with dogs and cats.

Corneal reflex and pupil size

The small animal placed under anesthesia should be very carefully touched along the lateral aspect of the cornea to stimulate the corneal reflex. If reflex closure of the eye does not occur with this stimulation, then the patient is moving into a deep plane 2 state and may be over-anesthetized. Minimize use of this reflex test to avoid injury to the cornea. Other monitoring devices should be more frequently relied on. The patient can be determined to be in a light, nonsurgical plane of anesthesia when the patient's pupils do not dilate. The patient's pupils will spontaneously constrict when a light, surgical plane has been reached. It is in the deeper, more intense plane of anesthesia (i.e., plane 3) that the patient's pupils again dilate. However, there are other factors that can induce dilation of the patient's pupils. These include the early "excitement" phase response to a preanesthetic medication or anesthesia, sympathetic responses to pain, or other drug-induced responses.

Pedal reflex and jaw tone

Another way to evaluate the depth of anesthesia is to check for the pedal reflex. This requires the technician to firmly squeeze (i.e., modestly pinch) the patient's skin— specifically, between the toes in dogs and cats, squeezing together the claws in cattle and swine, or applying firm pressure on the pastern of a horse. This action stimulates the animal's pedal reflex. The usual reaction is for the animal to pull the leg away. However, if properly anesthetized, the anesthetic plane greatly reduces the animal's response and reaction time. There are times when this response will disappear entirely. Patients considered to be within a surgical plane will not be able to respond to the stimulus at all.

The jaw tone or muscle tone of the animal can also be tested to determine the animal's depth of sedation. The test is conducted by grasping the lower jaw of the animal and attempting to open the animal's mouth widely, up to 3 times. This test is given to the animal prior to endotracheal intubation. The animal will usually resist the mouth-opening efforts. However, the anesthetic puts the patient into a very deep sleep, sufficient for the resistance response to dwindle. This response fades away to nothing when the animal reaches a light surgical plane. However, there are occasions when the addition of a strong analgesic or methoxyflurane can produce some signs of response. This does not indicate that a suitable plane of anesthesia has not been reached.

Heart rate, pulse rate, and rhythm

The heart rate should be carefully monitored during general anesthetic procedures. It is best to use a stethoscope to obtain an accurate assessment. Mechanical monitoring equipment with a digital readout can also be employed. Canines given anesthesia should have a heart rate ranging from 70 to 140 beats per minute. Felines given anesthesia should have a heart rate ranging from 100 to 140 beats per minute. The animal's heart rate may slow down when the anesthetic plane deepens in the patient. However, sometimes this may not be the case. Bradycardia can be caused by a number of drugs, as well as end-stage hypoxia and vagal nerve stimulation. In such situations the heart may still maintain a constant rate even when the patient falls into a dangerously deep state of anesthesia. Bradycardia can also be caused by hypotension. The pulse rate can be obtained by feeling the pulse along its artery. Pulse deficits are defined as diversions between the actual heartbeat and a palpable pulse response. These pulse response deficits must be recorded on the patient's chart. Arterial palpation and electrocardiograms should be used together to monitor the patient for arrhythmias. The electrocardiogram is the most precise device used.

Blood pressure and respiratory system

The peripheral pulse should be palpated with a gentle pressure to determine any increases or decreases in the beats. However, palpation cannot be used to come up with the actual cardiac and vascular performance values associated with the peripheral pulse. Commercially purchased, indirect or direct arterial blood pressure monitoring systems will give a more accurate measurement of blood pressure. Normal readings for blood pressure are: 100 to 160 mm Hg for the systolic, 80 to 120 mm Hg for the mean arterial, and 60 to 100 mm Hg for the diastolic. In most cases, the animal will be in deeper anesthetic planes when exhibiting a drop in blood pressure. Canines generally maintain a minimum level of 60 mm Hg for their mean blood pressures. Blood pressure can rise with hypercapnia (high levels of blood carbon dioxide, usually due to hypoventilation). However, blood pressure may sometimes be reduced with hypercapnia. Thus, the animal's rate and depth of the ventilation must be carefully monitored.

Capillary refill and mucous membrane color time

The capillary refill time is abbreviated as CRT. It is calculated as the amount of time it takes for blood flow to come back to an area after digital compression has been applied to an unpigmented mucous membrane (gingival tissue is a common site). The normal CRT is measured at less than 2 seconds. During general anesthesia, the CRT levels also require observation. In addition, the patient's blood pressure should be monitored concurrently. Blood pressure and CRT levels are both indicative of the quality of peripheral perfusion arising from cardiac output. CRT indices are expected to become more protracted as the anesthetic plane deepens and if hypovolemia (blood loss) ensues in the patient.

Unpigmented areas of mucous membrane are seen as pink when in a normal state. The discoloration of these tissues can be attributed to lower O2 levels. At such times the mucous membranes may change to the gray or blue coloration common to cyanosis. This transformation can be rapid or it may be delayed. A brilliant pink coloration can be attributed to the condition known as hypoventilation. This vasodilated color is the result of high CO_2 levels within the body caused by incomplete respiration and/or CO_2 retention.

Temperature

When the patient's metabolism slows down, the demand for anesthesia sufficient to maintain the surgical plane lessens as well. This is also true when the body temperature is reduced. Thus, the vital signs and body temperature should be carefully watched to prevent any complications from occurring during the procedure. The patient may require additional body temperature support when the anesthesia is first introduced into the body. This support may also be required during the recovery period. A digital thermometer can be used to monitor the axilla, peripheral, or rectal temperature of the animal. An esophageal temperature probe can be employed to find the animal's core temperature. Patients suffering with hypothermia require a warming treatment. This treatment is given to warm the body to 37.5 °C or 99 °F. Hyperthermia is avoided by terminating the heating support when the body reaches the correct temperature. The body can be warmed with hot water bottles or by way of BAIR hugger machines.

Stages of anesthesia

Stage I of anesthesia encompasses initial anesthetic administration up to the point of the loss of consciousness. This is known as the stage of induction, early analgesia, and altered state of consciousness. The patient may experience the following: dulled sensations, pain loss, blood pressure elevation, vomiting, inspiratory struggling, and coughing. The patient's pupils will begin to dilate as Stage II approaches. The patient's breathing rate is usually high and irregular at this time. Stage II commences with the loss of consciousness. In Stage II, the patient may experience the following: delirious activity and sounds, symptoms of involuntary struggling, and physiological agitation and excitement. During this time it is expected that the patient's eyes will remain closed and its jaw will be set. The patient's point reflexes may be amplified. The patient's pupils will be dilated and respond to light. Stage II does not last long.

Patients experiencing fairly uncomplicated inductions can move from stage I to stage III (the "surgical" stage) without incidence. Should the patient experience prolonged apnea, cardiac arrest, and/or brainstem or medullary paralysis, the "overdose" or fourth stage of the anesthesia will have been encountered and prompt remedial steps must immediately be taken. The third stage of anesthesia is maintained during the actual surgery. During this stage the patient's pupils will constrict further and the patient will gradually lose its palpebral (blink) reflex. However, the patient's breathing will be full and regular.

There are 4 planes associated with Stage III anesthesia. In plane 1 of Stage III, the patient retains its capacity to blink its eyes. The patient also retains its swallowing reflexes, and should be able to produce regular respirations with a respectable measure of chest activity. The patient will no longer be able to blink in plane 2 of Stage III, but will demonstrate a fixed pupil response. Respirations will continue to be regular and the chest and muscles in the diaphragm will continue to exhibit a good amount of movement. Plane 2, stage III is appropriate for the surgery executed by veterinarians. In plane 3 of stage III, the patient's breathing becomes shallow. This is due to a partial intercostal paralysis, limiting the patient's ability to breathe with its chest and abdominal muscles. In plane 4 of stage III, the patient enters an unstable and potentially life-threatening stage that should be avoided. This stage is formally reached when the patient ceases to breathe.

Analgesics

Analgesics given for anesthetic purposes require attention to the following factors: the timing of administration, the length of analgesia required, and the route of administration. A patient in pain can have some of its symptoms reduced with the application of an analgesic. This medication should not only reduce the animal's pain, but its anxiety as well. This can provide an easier preanesthetic and induction period for the pain-racked patient and for those laboring to render treatment. The amount of induction or maintenance agents needed may be lessened when analgesics are given to the patient preoperatively. The patient that is in the recovery period should continue to be given analgesics following a surgical procedure. The goal of the medication is to reduce the patient's stress and postoperative pain. Carefully administered analgesics are beneficial in reducing the patient's pain without rendering the patient unconscious. In this way the patient will remain in a more relaxed, responsive, and recovery-conducive state, where appropriate medications continue to alleviate the pain.

NSAIDS

Nonsteroidal anti-inflammatory drugs are abbreviated as NSAIDs. These drugs include the following: aspirin, acetaminophen, carprofen, ketoprofen, and meloxicam. These drugs are not dangerous to use in combination with opioids. NSAIDs are appropriate for the treatment of musculoskeletal pain. They are frequently applied in the treatment of patients with arthritis and other joint diseases. However, long-term NSAID therapy should not be used by patients with chronic kidney problems. The use of NSAIDs by this population can result in nephrotoxicity. It is best to use meloxicam in long-term therapy for renal-compromised patients, as has a lower risk for nephrotoxic results.

It is never appropriate to administer acetaminophen to a cat. Dogs should only be given acetaminophen on atypical occasions. Analgesics that are considered strong and safe can be given in direct postoperative orthopedic procedures. Pain medications are also particularly beneficial in the treatment of painful degloving injuries (where a large section of skin is severed from its underlying blood supply). Alternative medications include ketoprofen and carprofen.

Muscle relaxants

Neuromuscular blocking agents are employed during a surgical procedure to bring the patient into a state of more complete relaxation. The muscle relaxants have a number of beneficial effects. The positive effects include the following: an increase in the ability to manipulate the joints and bones, an improved contact and observation of the region being operated on, greater ease in regulating ventilation, easier endotracheal intubation, and the elimination of any residual eye movement in ocular surgical procedures. Muscle relaxants are particularly beneficial for those occasions when the patient cannot be subjected to a substantial amount of a deep anesthetic. In these cases, the patient experiences a reduction in the quantity of anesthetic agent required in the patient's treatment, and muscle relaxant adjuvants will enhance the surgical outcome and experience. A muscle relaxant–assisted surgical procedure should be conducted with the patient receiving constant ventilation. The patient should continue to be checked to determine the depth of anesthesia the patient is experiencing, with adjustments made accordingly.

Depth of anesthesia and ventilation

A muscle relaxant–assisted surgery will mask some of the usual signs used to monitor depth of anesthesia. Thus, regularly checking the depth of anesthesia takes on additional importance. Further, the patient will need another type of analgesic to reduce the pain. There are a multitude of neuromuscular blocking agents (muscle relaxants) that can be employed in patient care, including succinylcholine, gallamine, pancuronium, atracurium, and vecuronium. When such agents are employed, ventilation must be regulated by manual or mechanical means. One form of mechanical ventilation is referred to as intermittent positive pressure ventilation or IPPV. It involves establishing a preset respiratory rate.

Successful ventilation can help preserve normal acid-base levels by oxygenating the patient and reducing CO_2 retention. Assisted ventilation is usually necessary for overweight patients, patients in head-down recumbency, and patients with hypothermia or pulmonary disease. Ventilation is controlled with patients that receive neuromuscular blocking agents. In addition, patients with thoracic surgery, diaphragmatic hernia, gastric torsion, or hypoventilation should receive this same care. The veterinarian should note the respiratory rate, inspiration-to-expiration ratio, tidal volume, and inspiratory pressure. These outcomes should be reassessed continuously throughout the surgery. Ventilation is further checked by looking at the animal's chest motions arising from the breathing process.

The use of assisted ventilation predisposes the delivery of additional anesthetic to the patient. Thus, the patient will require a reduction in the percentage of delivered inhalant anesthetic at this juncture. The patient that demonstrates spontaneous breathing while receiving IPPV is being underventilated. Overventilation is not advisable, as it can cause the pulmonary alveoli to be harmed.

The patient in an underventilated state will have a reduced cardiac output. Respiratory alkalosis can be a result of unwarranted levels of CO_2. The patient with pneumothorax requires careful treatment. The danger of a collapsed lung is a strong possibility. The patient should receive continued ventilatory support for a few minutes after the inhalant anesthetic is turned off. This additional ventilatory support will be essential to the patient's speedy recovery. This directly assists in ridding the body of residual inhalant anesthetic.

Replacement fluids for stable anesthetic cases

The sedated and stable patient can be given IV fluid replacement crystalloids like Normosol R or Plasmalyte 148. Maintenance crystalloids include Normosol M or Plasmalyte 56. Replacement crystalloids are comparable to plasma because they have high sodium and chloride levels with a reduced potassium concentration. These medications can be administered according to the following general formula: 5 to 10 mL/kg/hr. Longer applications will require that the first hour be run at 10 mL/kg/hr, with additional hours reduced to 5 mL/kg/hr. The patient that loses fluids should receive supplemental fluids. This includes patients that have need for replacement of blood lost. The medical staff should be prepared to act in case of an emergency when a patient receives IV fluids. The medical staff will adhere to patent IV standards in this administration of IV fluids.

Respiratory acidosis

Respiratory acidosis is a result of CO_2 excretion that is lower than the CO_2 produced. An escalation of CO_2 levels in the blood gases can be attributed to this situation. Conditions that contribute to hypoventilation include: a state of deep anesthesia, pulmonary disease, or respiratory obstruction. Reduced ventilation is also responsible for CO_2 retention. These circumstances can bring about respiratory acidosis. Patients that have a more concentrated level of CO_2 will more than likely have a lower pH level. Thus, the patient's acid levels will rise as the CO_2 builds. Cardiac outputs will also rise in patients with hypertension. This condition points to respiratory acidosis. In addition, vasodilatation or ventricular arrhythmias can also suggest respiratory acidosis. The body is able to compensate for this circumstance with time. Initially, the body releases acid buffers. In 3-5 days, kidney excretion of carbonic acid rises as does bicarbonate reabsorption. Respiratory acidosis can be treated by ventilatory volume and by treating the underlying disease that caused the higher levels of carbon dioxide.

Respiratory alkalosis

Respiratory alkalosis is a result of a patient's excreting more CO_2 than is produced. Lower levels of CO_2 in blood gas analyses point to this condition. This may occur as a result of mechanical respiratory hyperventilation. It can also be caused by spontaneous hyperventilation in patients suffering from extreme pain or some other source of overstimulation. Lower levels of CO_2 will produce lower quantities of acids and drive an increase in basic pH. The patient suffering from respiratory alkalosis may exhibit tachycardia and other electrocardiographic anomalies. The kidneys may be able to counteract the effects, if given enough time. Further, a mechanically ventilated patient can be given a lower minute volume of ventilation to reduce the effects of respiratory alkalosis. Hyperventilation should be addressed by the medical staff.

Metabolic acidosis

Metabolic acidosis can be attributed to a low adjusted base excess. The low adjusted base excess can be written as ABE. Metabolic acidosis can also be a result of low HCO3- — as confirmed by blood gas analysis. Metabolic acidosis can also be brought on by lactic acid gain, renal failure, and losing and not reabsorbing HCO3-rich body secretions. Diarrhea can also lead to this problematic condition. Higher levels of H+ can be detected when HCO3- is lost. Hyperventilation can produce a natural relief to this problem. An alkalinizing IV solution can also be administered to the patient to correct a minor imbalance. Sodium bicarbonate can be administered to patients to restore more acute imbalances. However, this can be a deadly approach for patients suffering from dehydration. In this situation the patient would be suffering from 2 disorders. However, one is considered the primary disorder. The other is a secondary disorder which contributes to the primary problem. The blood gas results should be noted and interpreted according to the factors associated with both the primary and secondary disorders.

Interpretation of blood gases

The veterinarian should always monitor a patient's pH levels. These levels should range from 7.35 to 7.45. Lower rates of pH are indicative of acidosis. Higher rates are indicative of alkalosis. The PCO2 can also be used to determine the patient's respiratory condition. The ABE (adjusted base excess) levels can be used to determine the patient's metabolic condition. The primary disorder will be the one that produces the most change in the patient. The patient's pH can be indicative of the direction in which the changes are taking place. The metabolic state is determined by the ABE levels, despite the presence of irregular levels of CO2. This can be attributed to the changes in PCO2 that are assessed along with the ABE level. Normal levels of CO2 suggest that the metabolic state can be determined through analysis of the HCO3-. Metabolic acidosis can be detected when HCO3- is less than 20. However, levels over 26 imply metabolic alkalosis exists.

Oxygenation and anesthetic equipment problems

Some problems associated with anesthetic delivery can be traced to mechanical dysfunction. The problem can be as simple as a disconnected endotracheal tube, rebreathing bag, or breathing hose. The problem may also be found in leaking or blocked equipment. These issues can contribute to the poor oxygenation of a patient. Sometimes such a problem will lead directly to medication overdosing or under-dosing. For example, anesthesia under-administration may be traced to an empty vaporizer. A broken or ineffective setting on a vaporizer can also cause this problem. In addition, sometimes the problem is found in hoses that are not securely fastened, poorly connecting the patient to the device.

Too much carbon dioxide can be the result of an exhausted CO2 absorbant or a stuck unidirectional valve. Sometimes, the mixture of anesthesia administered to a patient may be in a hypoxic form. This happens when the nitrous oxide levels are too high when matched with the O2 flow. The higher settings on the vaporizer can result in a patient that has been over-anesthetized. The patient may then suffer from acute hypercapnia or hypoxia. Consequently, all mechanical equipment must be examined prior to use, and maintained regularly.

Anatomy/Physiology/Parasitology

Cells

Prokaryotic cells are simple organisms without a nucleus (i.e., a central structure that contains chromosomes and genes). Bacteria are a common form of prokaryotes. A typical bacterium is a single celled, parasitic microorganism. Bacteria are parasitic in that they live in or on and feed off of other organisms. Eukaryotic cells are characterized by multiple complex structures enclosed within cellular membranes. Most eukaryotes have 3 main parts. The first part is the outer cell membrane or protective shell that allows oxygen and food particles to pass through, and waste to be excreted. The second part is the inner cytoplasm – an organic compound with the consistency of jelly – that contains cytosol and organelles. In animal life, cytoplasm occupies over half of the cell's volume. Cytosol is the watery portion of the cytoplasm, excluding all structures and organelles. Cellular organelles, such as mitochondria, chloroplasts, and Golgi bodies, perform specific functions within the cell. The third part of the eukaryotic cell, also found in the cytoplasm, is the nucleus. It contains genetic material and controls cell growth and reproduction processes.

There are numerous organelles found in cellular cytoplasm. They include ribosomes, mitochondria, endoplasmic reticula, chloroplasts (chlorophyll, in plant cells), and Golgi bodies. Ribosomes are cellular organelles which manufacture cellular proteins. They can be found freely floating in the cytoplasm, arranged in small clusters, or attached to endoplasmic reticula (intracellular tubular membranes which transport materials). Ribosomes manufacture essential proteins by "reading" the RNA produced by genetic DNA, and translating it into the kind of protein indicated. Mitochondria are specialized organelles which make up as much as 25% of the cytoplasm. Mitochondria transform organic substances from foods into a useable source of chemical energy. The endoplasmic reticulum is a network of tubes that alters and transports proteins, produces and stores macromolecules (i.e., glycogen and natural steroids), and sequesters calcium. Golgi bodies process cellular products, releasing them back into the cell or excreting them as needed.

The cytoskeleton is the framework of the cell, and allows movement within the cell. Further, this structure protects the cell. Intracellular transportation is carried out as organelles and vesicles move about within the cytoskeleton framework.

Within each cell is a "center" called the centrosome. It organizes cellular microtubules, and regulates cell-cycle progression. Within the centrosome are centrioles. Centrioles organize and replicate the mitotic spindle for successful cell division and reorganization. The Golgi complex (also called the Golgi body, apparatus, or dictyosome) serves as a processing and routing system for the cell. This organelle packages proteins for use in the cell or for secretion outside the cell. The Golgi complex also builds lysosomes, which are responsible for breaking down and recycling molecules within the cell. Non-working organelles, intracellular bacteria, lipids, carbohydrates, and proteins are also contained in the lysosomes.

Arising from the endoplasmic reticulum are "peroxisomes," which are responsible for removing toxins from the cell. Peroxisome enzymes known as oxidase and catalase carry out this elimination process. Peroxisomes can self-replicate through a process of enlarging and division.

Tissue

There are 4 primary tissue types in the human body: epithelial, connective, muscle, and nerve tissue. Epithelial tissue lines the exterior of the body, as well as all cavities and surfaces of solid structures within the body. This tissue is composed of either a single-cell layer (i.e., simple squamous or columnar cells) or several "stratified" layers of cells. Primary epithelial tissue functions include: secretion, excretion, absorption, protection, sensation detection, and selective permeability.

The second type of tissue is known as connective tissue. This tissue is located in a variety of places within the body. Connective tissue types determine the function that is carried out. Some types of connective tissues work to connect, support, and protect the structures and organs within the body. Other types of connective tissues work to insulate. Still others are responsible for the transportation of fluids and for energy storage.

Muscle tissue consists of 3 main subtypes known as skeletal, smooth, and cardiac muscle. Skeletal muscle is described as striated contractile tissue attached to the skeleton. It has a striated appearance – characterized by alternating light and dark bands under microscopic view. Skeletal muscle is responsible for voluntary control and movement. Smooth muscle is involuntarily controlled muscle, and is found in the walls of the hollow organs. It moves much more slowly, has no striations, and is "autonomically" or involuntarily regulated. Hollow organs, specifically, blood vessels, bladder, uterus, and the gastrointestinal tract derive dilation, contraction, and peristaltic movement from smooth muscles. The third muscle tissue subtype, Cardiac muscle, is located within the heart. It is also striated, but unlike striated skeletal muscle, it is involuntarily controlled.

The fourth type of tissue is nervous tissue. It is located within the brain, spinal cord, and nerves. Neurons and neuroglia are 2 key cell types. Neurons are nerve cells which work to transmit signals or impulses, to react to stimuli, or produce voluntary actions or responses. Neuroglia (or "glial") cells can be described as a network of tissues and fibers found in the brain and spinal column that provide support, protection, and nutrition to neurons, among other functions.

Bone

Types
The 2 major types of bone are compact bone and cancellous (also called "trabecular" or "spongy") bone. Compact bones give structural strength and support to the body. Compact bones allow for strenuous movement and weight-bearing activities. Compact bone is composed of very tightly grouped osteons (also called "haversian systems"). Each osteon is

comprised of a solid matrix of osseous lamellae (concentric rings of deposited minerals and proteins) surrounding a central canal containing blood vessels to nurture the bone. Between the lamellar rings are osteocytes (bone cells) situated in lacunae (small spaces). Channels called canaliculi extend from the lacunae to the osteonic (or haversian) canal. Nutrition is brought in through the canaliculi, and waste is moved out.

Cancellous bone is found inside and at the rounded ends of long bones, in the pelvic bones and breastbone. Its primary purpose is to protect bone marrow, and to provide interior structural support. Cancellous bone is honeycomb-like in appearance, having numerous cavities and spaces interspersed with boney plates and ridges known as trabeculae. Trabeculae are arranged to provide maximum support for stresses and loads incurred, and may gradually rearrange themselves in response to new stresses or burdens. Cancellous bone does not receive nourishment via osteonic canals (i.e., haversian systems), but rather via canaliculi connecting the various spaces within the trabecular structure. Osseous trabeculae may be composed of mineralized bone or collagen. Collagen is a connective tissue made up of fibrous proteins. The larger trabecular spaces are filled with red bone marrow, where the production of blood cellular components takes place.

Classifications

Bones are typically classified by shape, often using 4 categories: long, short, flat, and irregular. However, other classification systems use 6 categories: long, short, flat, pneumatic, sesamoid, and irregular (or "sutural"). Using the 6-category classification system, the first bone type is the long bones. Long bones grow primarily through a lengthening of the diaphysis (shaft). The diaphysis is the midsection of the long bone. The diaphysis has 2 rounded ends which are called epiphyses. The long bone also has a marrow cavity, also called a medullar cavity. The medullar cavity is the central section of bone where the yellow bone marrow is kept. Two examples of long bones are the radius and the femur. The radius in most animals is found in the lower forelimb. The femur in most animals is the upper rear leg bone, and is typically the strongest bone in the body.

The second type of the 6 classifications of bones refers to the short bones. The short bones share some similar structural characteristics found in the long bones. However, the short bones do not have a medullar cavity in which to house yellow bone marrow. Short bone examples include the boney digits within the hand and fingers. The third type of the 6 classification system of bones includes the flat bones, which are thin, level, horizontal bones. Flat bones are formed from 2 layers of compact bone with a middle layer of cancellous bone. The skull bones, ribs, pelvis, and scapula are all classified as flat bones. The fourth type of the classification system includes the pneumatic bones. Pneumatic bones have an air-filled cavity or indentation, such as that found in the sinuses. The fifth type includes the sesamoid bones. Sesamoid bones are small, short bones of an irregular spherical or sesame seed–like shape. The sesamoid bone helps to alleviate some of the stress caused by friction, and/or to reduce pressures otherwise applied to a tendon or joint. One example of a sesamoid bone is the patella or kneecap. The sixth type includes the irregular bones. Irregular bones are bones that do not fit into the classifications of long bones, short bones, flat bones, pneumatic bones, or sesamoid bones.

Copyright © Mometrix Media. You have been licensed one copy of this document for personal use only. Any other reproduction or redistribution is strictly prohibited. All rights reserved.

Central nervous system

The brain is the organ within the body that has control over the central nervous system. In its most elemental form, the central nervous system consists of the brain and the spinal cord. The brain itself consists of the cerebrum (the 2 hemispheres that collectively make up the forebrain and midbrain), the cerebellum (or "small brain"), and the brain stem (connecting the brain and spinal cord). During embryological development, the emerging brain (existing then as 3 swellings in the embryonic neural tube) is divided into the prosencephalon, the mesencephalon, and the rhombencephalon. The prosencephalon becomes the forebrain, the mesencephalon becomes the midbrain, and the rhombencephalon becomes the hindbrain. The brain stem is the lower portion of the brain that is attached to the spinal cord.

The spinal cord is comprised of a thick cord of nerve cells that is attached to the bottom of the brain, or the brain stem. The spinal cord has a protective boney covering which is known as the vertebral column. The vertebral column is a part of the skeletal axis. The spinal cord sends out nerve impulses or signals by way of efferent nerve paths, and receives them by way of afferent nerve paths. Thus, afferent nerves transmit signals or sensory impulses to the central nervous system, while efferent nerves send impulses or signals away from the brain to the organs or muscles.

Additional features
The meninges are 3 layers of membranes which function to protect the central nervous system. The meninges are dense, fibrous connective tissues that enclose the spinal cord and the brain. The 3 layers are known as the dura mater, the arachnoid mater, and the pia mater.

Cerebrospinal fluid is a clear, water-like fluid found in and around the brain and the spinal cord. The cerebrospinal fluid works to cushion the central nervous system from pressures or outside forces. The cerebrospinal fluid is also a source of nourishment for the brain. The fluid contains essential protein, glucose, ions, and other substances that keep the central nervous system healthy and fit.

The blood-brain barrier (BBB) refers to certain extra-dense membranes lining the capillaries of the brain. This barrier allows certain liquids or substances to pass through to the central nervous system while preventing the entrance of many others. It is yet another form of protection for the brain. Blood contains oxygen, glucose, and fat-soluble compounds that are able to pass through the blood-brain barrier. However, the blood-brain barrier keeps out waste products and many drugs.

Cardiac cycle

The cardiac cycle refers to all cardiac events that occur from one heartbeat to the next. The heart rate is largely determined by the demand for oxygen throughout the body – although arousal, stress, anxiety, and other factors may also intervene. The cardiac cycle may be divided into 2 phases: diastole and systole. A four-phase cycle is also sometimes described. Phase 1 is the ventricular filling period, occurring when the ventricles are in diastole. At this time the atria are in contraction, filling the ventricles. Phase 2 is the isovolumetric contraction period, which begins with ventricular systole initiation. Phase 3 is the ventricular ejection period, when the ventricles contract and send blood into the pulmonary artery and aorta. The fourth and final phase is the isovolumetric relaxation period, initiated upon ventricular return to diastole.

Hematic oxygenation response

The oxygenation of blood is completed by way of the cardiac cycle, through the heart's 4 chambers. The right atrium is the part of the heart that accepts deoxygenated blood from the superior and inferior vena cava. The vena cava is the largest vein that carries blood back to the heart. From the right atrium, deoxygenated blood is sent into the right ventricle. The right ventricle then contracts, moving the deoxygenated blood into the lungs. The lungs are responsible for the diffusion of carbon dioxide out of the blood in exchange for oxygen diffusion into the bloodstream, as gaseous molecular equilibrium is obtained. The oxygenated blood then flows out of the lungs and into the left atrium. The left atrium is the upper left chamber of the heart. Once filled with oxygenated blood the left atrium contracts, sending the blood into the left ventricle, where its contraction forces the blood out and into the aorta. From that point, the oxygenated blood moves throughout the body's arteries and then veins to complete the hematic response to the cardiac cycle.

Vascular system

Blood vessels

Blood is the red body fluid that flows within the body's vascular system. Blood is carried by a system of vessels or tubular channels. Arterial vessels carry oxygenated blood away from the heart, and venous vessels carry deoxygenated blood to the heart. The pulmonary vein is unique in that it is responsible for carrying oxygenated blood to the heart from the lungs. Oxygenated blood is blood that has been combined with oxygen, and from which carbon dioxide has been removed. The blood is moved under pressure from the heart. Artery walls are thicker than the walls of veins, as they must sustain direct cardiac pumping pressures. However, on average, veins are larger in diameter and have many one-way valves to facilitate the passive return process. Larger arteries divide into smaller blood vessels known as arterioles. The arterioles distribute blood from the arteries to the capillaries. The force of blood applied at regular intervals by way of cardiac contraction is known as blood pressure.

Capillary and venous return features

Capillaries have walls that are constructed from a single layer of endothelium. This allows the exchange of carbon dioxide and oxygen gases by molecular diffusion, as well as the osmotic exchange of nutrient fluids and waste molecules (such as glucose and urea) via the capillary stream. Capillaries are described as the smallest blood vessels found in the body. They also serve as a depressurizing link between the arteries and veins in the body.

Veins are described as any blood vessel that transports deoxygenated blood within the body (with the exception of the pulmonary vein, which carries oxygenated blood back to the heart). Venous walls are much thinner than arterial walls, as they accommodate a much lower blood pressure than that of the arteries. Veins have interspersing one-way valves as an essential feature, to prevent any backflow of deoxygenated blood. Backflow could otherwise be caused by low blood pressures in the body. Venules are the venous counterpart to arterioles, and carry blood back to larger venous vessels.

Digestion

Digestion is a process that food undergoes so that the body can absorb and use its nutrients. The digestive process terminates in the excretion of waste. The digestive process uses certain substances which can chemically change food into nutrients that the body can absorb. The digestive process incorporates both mechanical and chemical actions in the breakdown and absorption of food. The mouth is the starting point in the digestive process.

Food enters the mouth to be ground up into smaller particles before being swallowed. It is in the mouth that food is first combined with digestive enzymes (such as salivary amylase) as it is chewed or masticated. Digestive enzymes work to further break down the food. The esophagus carries the food down to the stomach. There, the food is mixed with additional digestive enzymes known as gastric juices. Gastric juices are formed from hydrochloric acid, protein-digesting enzymes, and mucus. More youthful stomachs may also contain the proteolytic enzyme chymosin (also called rennin). Chymosin is used to coagulate milk, converting it from a liquid into a semisolid mass.

After being acted upon by the gastric juices, ingested food becomes a softened, semi-solid mass called chyme. Chyme is described as a combination of water, hydrochloric acid, and digestive enzymes. Chyme is passed from the stomach into the small intestine. The small intestine is responsible for a major portion of the digestion and absorption process. The small intestine is located between the stomach and the large intestine. The small intestine releases pancreatic and intestinal enzymes to be blended with the chyme. Gradually the chyme is separated by the lacteals into chyle (emulsified fats and fatty acids) and excrement. The chyle is taken up by the lacteals and passed into the lymphatic system. From there it is transported into the bloodstream via the thoracic duct. The excrement travels from the small intestine into the large intestine, where excess water is absorbed. The latter part of the small intestine (the ilium) and the large intestine are host to considerable bacteria, many of which act to synthesize niacin (nicotinic acid), thiamin (vitamin B1), and vitamin K, which are then absorbed into the body. Finally, undigested food is transported to the rectum, located between the colon and the anal canal. The body releases this undigested food as feces, which passes through the anus.

Ruminant digestion
Ruminant digestion is a process of digestion used by animals with hooves. The animal eats raw, unprocessed material and then regurgitates or brings food up from the stomach in a form that has not been completely softened or digested. The food that is partially softened is referred to as a cud or bolus. The animal proceeds to further masticate the cud, which allows it to digest the material more thoroughly. This is known as remasticated food. Remasticated or chewed food continues to be mixed with a clear liquid known as saliva. The remasticated

food is then re-swallowed and split into layers of solid matter and liquid matter in the first 2 chambers of the stomach. This additional swallowing of food is known as deglutition. The first 2 chambers of the stomach are known as the rumen and the reticulum. The ruminant stomach actually contains 4 compartments in total, called the rumen, the reticulum, the omasum, and the abomasum. The abomasum is referred to as the "true" or glandular stomach, as it is where final acidic and enzymatic digestion takes place.

The rumen (the first stomach chamber) is the most spacious of all the chambers in the ruminant animal. The rumen is responsible for blending the food with the right amount of pH, temperature, and bacteria in anaerobic conditions. The second chamber is known as the reticulum or the second stomach. Cows and sheep have this type of stomach. The lining of this compartment has a hexagonal honeycomb pattern. This pattern is beneficial to the process of absorption. Absorption through this expansive surface area allows for the taking in of volatile fatty acids.

The omasum is the third chamber in the ruminant stomach, and is responsible for further crushing of food. The omasum absorbs or soaks up water, magnesium, and bicarbonate. The omasum is located between the reticulum and the abomasum. The abomasum is the fourth stomach on a ruminant animal. This is the true stomach, as it is responsible for blending the food with digestive enzymes. This blending causes chemical digestion to begin. The chemical digestion allows nutrients to be absorbed by the small intestine.

Ear

The ear is the organ responsible for hearing and balance in mammals. The ear has 3 main parts: the outer ear, middle ear, and the inner ear. The outer ear includes the pinna (the visible outside ear or auricle), the auditory canal, and the tympanic membrane or eardrum. The middle ear transmits sound from the outer ear to the inner ear via 3 articulating bones called ossicles. The ossicles are named as follows: 1) the malleus or hammer, 2) the incus or anvil, and 3) the stapes or stirrup. Each bone is nicknamed in both Latin and English according to its shape. The small bones vibrate to amplify and relay sound waves from the eardrum to the inner ear. The Eustachian tube links the middle ear to the nasal cavity. The liquid in the inner ear helps maintain balance. The inner ear consists of the cochlea and the semicircular canals. The cochlea is coiled in shape like a snail shell. The cochlea has thousands of hair cells that move in response to sound waves, generating auditory nerve impulses in response. The "organ of Corti," the principal section of the cochlea, translates the neural impulses into sounds. The sound transmission is conducted by an impulse that makes its way from the brain along the auditory nerve.

Whole blood

Whole blood is made up of fluid and cellular substances that join to carry out specific functions within the body. One of the fluids is called plasma. Plasma has a very light yellowish color. Plasma is the primary liquid in which hematic cells are dispersed to form whole blood. Plasma is 90% water and 10% blood plasma proteins. There are also traces of other materials in this substance. The hematic cells in whole blood each have a specific function within the body. Erythrocytes, leukocytes, and thrombocytes make up the cellular components in whole blood. The substance in the plasma that is responsible for clotting is known as fibrinogen protein. Removal of fibrinogen protein leaves a fluid substance known as serum. Blood is a necessary component in the body. Blood transports dissolved proteins, oxygen, carbon dioxide, hormones, lipids, and metabolic end products within the body. The blood flows within the circulatory system as the heart pumps blood to the lungs and then throughout the body.

Urinary excretory system

The excretory system is a complex network that discharges waste materials left over from the metabolic functions of the body. The body can expel waste through the action of defecating or urinating. The urinary excretory system is made up of the kidneys, ureters, urinary bladder, and the urethra. The kidneys remove liquid waste from the bloodstream. This liquid waste is called urine, which is expelled from the body.

Each species of animal has a specific shaped and sized kidney, although most are shaped in the form of a bean. The ureters are urinary ducts responsible for transporting urine away from the kidneys and into the bladder in mammals. The ureter is fashioned from smooth muscle. The urinary bladder is a hollow, stretchy sac used for urine storage. Urine is collected and stored until it is discharged. Urine ultimately passes through the urethra, which is a tube extending from the bladder to the body's exterior. The urethra is fashioned from smooth muscle, with a sphincter between itself and the bladder that operates under voluntary control for this discharge process.

Urine production
The excretory system incorporates 3 phases in urinary production. The 3 phases are referred to as filtration, reabsorption, and secretion. The filtration phase occurs in one of the many nephrons found in the kidney. Within each nephron is a circular-shaped cluster of capillaries called the glomerulus. It resides under a thin, double-membraned outer covering called Bowman's capsule. High pressures from the renal artery force water, salt, and other small molecules out of the glomerulus. This solution of water, salt, and other molecules is known as glomerular filtrate. This solution is then filtered through Bowman's capsule. Bowman's capsule is responsible for removing waste products, inorganic salts, and excess water.

The second phase of urinary production occurs when nutrients that are left over from this filtration process are reabsorbed into the body through renal tubules. Principally, this reabsorption is carried out in the proximal convoluted tubules or PCTs, with reabsorbed materials entering the surrounding peritubular capillaries. The process of concentrating and absorbing salts is carried out in the nephron tubule known as the loop of Henle. In the third phase of urinary production, blood pH is regulated in the distal convoluted tubules (DCTs) by processes of absorption and secretion, with certain substances released into the DCTs from the peritubular capillaries.

Bilirubin

Bilirubin is a brownish-yellow substance found in bile. It is the by-product of hemoglobin, released when aging or superfluous red blood cells are broken down by reticuloendothelial cells found in the liver, spleen, and bone marrow. Other chromoproteins may also contain heme and thus contribute to the formation of bilirubin when broken down. Bilirubin is responsible for the yellowish appearance in bruises, as well as the yellow, icteric appearance of the skin when jaundice develops – typically due to liver dysfunction. Bilirubin is formed by the metabolism of heme, which is the deep red iron-containing pigment found in the blood. As red blood cells die, they are broken down into heme and globins. Eventually the heme is changed into Fe^{2+}, carbon monoxide, and bilirubin.

Elevated bilirubin levels are common in newborns, as high numbers of red blood cells, needed only in the womb (due to low oxygen transfer through the placenta), are rapidly destroyed at birth. Bilirubin can become toxic in neonates, as the blood-brain barrier remains immature and may be unable to protect sensitive brain tissues from the deleterious effects of hyperbilirubinemia (jaundice). Bilirubin is rapidly broken down by light; thus newborns are assisted in the breakdown of bilirubin by being placed under special lighting for treatment.

In its primary form, bilirubin is unconjugated – i.e., not joined together with other substances. This unconjugated form of bilirubin is lipid-soluble and thus can readily attach itself to serum proteins. The resulting solution is transported to the liver for conjugation. The conjugated form of bilirubin is water-soluble, which means it can be dissolved completely in water. The conjugated form of bilirubin has the basic structure of glucuronic acid. Glucuronic acid is derived from glucose. The combination of glucuronic acid with drugs, pollutants, acids, and other toxins tends to render them harmless through a process known as glucuronidation. Glucuronidation is the body's way of producing water-soluble forms that can readily be discharged from the body through urination.

Finally, bilirubin can be used to check for hepatic (liver) damage. Evaluation involves the measurement of the amount of bilirubin that is present in the urine. Laboratory tests can measure total bilirubin, along with direct (conjugated) and indirect (unconjugated) levels. With a properly functioning liver, the bilirubin should virtually all be in a conjugated form. However, this is not true when hepatic (liver) damage is present. An excessive amount of unconjugated serum bilirubin indicates prehepatic jaundice or hepatic-induced jaundice. Likewise, this can be determined by the levels present in the urine.

Skeletal articulations

A skeletal articulation exists whenever 2 bones come together for purposes of movement. Another name for an articulation is a joint. A joint is structurally created when tissue binds 2 or more bones together. The tissue can consist of fibrous, elastic, or cartilaginous materials. Joints can be classified by way of the following kinds of articulations: synarthrosis, amphiarthrosis, and diarthrosis. Synarthrosis joints are fixed in a permanent position. An example can be seen in the suture joints of the skull. Amphiarthrosis joints allow only limited movement, such as the pubic symphysis. Symphysis indicates that the bones merge naturally. Diarthrosis refers to a joint that is capable of changing position in multiple of directions. An example would be the shoulder, which allows wide ranging motion.

There are 3 additional types of structural joint classifications: fibrous, cartilaginous, and synovial. The first 2 are classified according to the tissues creating the joint (fibers or cartilage). The last refers to the synovial fluid feature that characterizes this joint. Fibrous joints are bony articulations joined by strong fibers. These joints are intended to move little if at all. One example of fibrous joints can be seen in the skull sutures. The only time these joints move is during the process of birth, to accommodate the confines of the birth canal. However, they persist in fibrous form as points of subsequent cranial growth. In late adulthood they eventually fuse. Joints that are linked by cartilage without a joint cavity are known as cartilaginous joints. Cartilage is a strong, stretchy tissue. Cartilaginous joint examples include intervertebral discs and the pubic symphysis.

Synovial joints are identified by the presence of synovial fluid — a clear viscous fluid that provides the joint with lubrication and nourishment. These joints have a joint capsule or sac which contains synovial fluid. The synovial membrane (or bursa) is a thin layer of tissue that encloses both cartilaginous and non-cartilaginous surfaces, creating a joint capsule. The synovial membrane is responsible for the secretion of the synovial fluid. The limb joints found within the body are synovial joints. Synovial joints can also be diarthrotic joints.

Anatomical direction

There are 12 descriptive terms of anatomical direction. These terms can be grouped according to varying similarities in reference points. For example, a direction can be described in terms that indicate the location of the body part. Therefore, a direction toward the head is referred to as cranial. A direction toward the tail is known as caudal. The direction that refers to the backbone is called dorsal. The direction away from the backbone is known as ventral. The direction that describes the location nearest to the median plane is known as the medial. The direction that is the longest distance away from the median plane is known as the lateral. The location that is nearest to the backbone is called the proximal — used particularly when one is referring to the nearer aspect of limbs or appendages. The location farthest from the backbone is called distal — used particularly when one refers to the more distant aspect of limbs or appendages. The term anterior can be applied when one is talking about the direction of the head. The term posterior can be used when one is talking about the direction of the tail. The term palmar is used to describe the palm of the hand or bottom of a front foot, hoof, or paw. The term plantar is used to describe the area on the bottom of the foot, or rear hoof or paw.

Estrous cycle

Phases

The phases of the estrous cycle circumscribe the duration of time that a female mammal can exhibit signs of sexual receptivity that may attract a mate. During this period of time the female has reoccurring physiological changes that can be attributed to the effects of reproductive hormones. There are 4 estrous phases: proestrus, estrus, diestrus, and anestrus. Some schema include a fifth phase called metestrus, which is very brief (1-5 days) immediately following the estrus phase.

Proestrus is the time period just before onset the estrus cycle. The proestrus period is designed to prepare the uterus to receive an embryo. Follicle Stimulating Hormone or FSH induces ovarian follicles to develop and give off estrogen. Estrogen is a steroid hormone produced by the ovaries, which builds up in the uterus and uterine horns. During proestrus, estrogen induces endothelium to grow and form an inner layer in the uterus. This inside layer develops in preparation for a potentially fertilized egg to implant.

With the onset of estrus, the female is able to function in the reproductive process and ovulation occurs. The female's uterus and uterine horns are fully prepared to accept an embryo. Canines also experience a surge in luteinizing hormone (LH), which comes from the pituitary gland. The luteinizing hormone is responsible for ovulation, and indicates that the egg or eggs from the ovaries are ready for fertilization. Ovulation in cats and rabbits occurs through the breeding process, as they are nonspontaneous or induced ovulators.

A third phase called metestrus begins as luteinizing hormone levels begin to drop. In this post-ovulatory phase, each egg-containing follicle changes, bursts, and grows into a corpus luteum. A corpus luteum is a yellow mass that produces progesterone to continue thickening the lining of the uterus. The corpus luteum is needed to begin and to maintain a pregnancy, and functions to produce hormones during the next phase of the estrus cycle (diestrus). Finally, all sexual hormonal activity ceases during the concluding phase called anestrus (the resting phase).

Pregnancy

Pregnancy exists when a female animal carries an unborn offspring inside her body. A healthy pregnancy lasts from the time of fertilization to the birthing process. During the estrus cycle, the corpus luteum will work to consistently produce essential pregnancy- related hormones throughout most or all of a pregnancy. The duration of the production of hormone will vary in accordance with the type of species. Some types of animals will require the hormones to be produced throughout the entire period of the pregnancy. Other types of animals will only require the hormones until the placenta is formed. The placenta is a transient organ inside the uterus that pregnant female mammals produce to supply oxygen and food to a fetus. Nutrition, oxygen, and other substances are delivered to the fetus through the umbilical cord. The umbilical cord is a flexible tube that links the abdomen of the fetus to the mother's placenta. This tube is also used to expel waste. The intrauterine corpus luteum will break down or decompose if a pregnancy does not actualize (i.e., if a fertilized egg does not implant there).

Female reproductive system

The female reproductive system consists of many interrelated organs and anatomical features. The ovaries are a pair of organs necessary for female reproduction. The oval-shaped ovaries are located in the female's abdomen. Ovaries are responsible for the production of ova and hormones. The ova are female reproductive cells. Ova is a Latin word for "eggs," and the words may be used interchangeably. In most species, the ova will pass from the ovary to the uterine horn or uterus, down to the uterine tubes (or Fallopian tubes or oviduct). The uterus has the following parts: uterine horns, body, and cervix, leading to the opening of the uterus. Uterine horns are the projections from the uterus that extend toward the uterine or fallopian tubes. Some animals do not have uterine horns.
Some animals are polytocous or multiparous (which means that the animal is able to have more than one baby at a given time), and will typically have longer uterine horns in order to carry several offspring. The species that have only 1 baby are known as monotocous or uniparous. Their fetuses will grow & develop in the uterus itself. There are 3 layers within the uterus and uterine horns. These 3 layers are: endometrium, myometrium, and perimetrium. During the birthing process, the fetus will pass out of the uterus to the exterior environment. The vehicle for this passage is known as the vagina or birth canal. The vulva is the name given to the external female genitalia, which consists of the labia and opening to the urethra and internal sex organs.

Preservation of parasitic samples

There are a number of steps to take in the preservation of parasitic samples that will be sent away for diagnostic testing. It is essential that the sample be kept in an unchanged condition for accurate diagnostic confirmation. The first step requires that fresh samples be packed in leak-proof containers. These containers should be sealed securely. The containers with the fecal samples require a label with the following information: date, site from which the specimen was acquired, the animal owner's name, the species of the animal, an identification number for the animal and/or the name of the animal, the referring veterinarian, the address of the clinic, and the telephone number. The fecal sample can be sent for outside laboratory testing in its pure form. The fecal sample may also be mixed with a solution of 10% formalin at a ratio of 1:3. Formalin is a solution of formaldehyde in water. The use of a diluted alcohol or formalin solution is recommended to preserve whole parasites or segments of parasites for proper laboratory microscopic examination, identification, and relative concentration or "parasitic load" indices.

Modified Knott's technique

Modified Knott's technique is used to identify and name the blood parasites. There are many kinds of blood-borne parasites (commonly classified as: rickettsial, protozoal, helminth, and viral). Two types of blood parasites that infest dogs are the Dirofilaria immitis (dog

- 82 -

heartworm), and Dipetalonema reconditum. The latter can sometimes be mistaken for the former, but Dirofilaria is much more dangerous. The genus Dipetalonema has recently been reorganized, and the new name is Acanthocheilonema reconditum. However, use of the old name persists. The modified Knott's technique requires 15 mL centrifuge tube and centrifuge, 2% formalin solution, methylene blue stain, Pasteur pipettes and bulbs, and microscope slides and coverslips. A centrifuge tube is used for the sample of EDTA (anticoagulant) blood (1mL) and 2% formalin or water (9 mL). The solution disrupts the red blood cell's bonding membrane, causing it to "lyse" or burst. This mixture is placed in the centrifuge at 1000 rpm for 5 minutes. An alternative allows the solution to remain still for 1 hour. The supernatant or liquid on the surface is gently decanted off, so as not to disrupt the sediment. Next, 2 drops of methylene blue is applied to the undisturbed sediment. Aspirating gently with the pipette mixes the solution. A miniscule sample is positioned on a microscope slide and covered with a coverslip. The microscope is set at a ten-power objective. This setting is used to examine the entire slide for microfilariae or larva of an infesting parasite.

Parasitology

Identification of non-burrowing external parasitic mites

Parasites are those organisms which live on or in a host organism. Ectoparasites live on the surface of the host, and include fleas, ticks, lice, and mites. Endoparasites live inside the animal, and include heartworms, roundworms, hookworms, lungworms, whipworms, and tapeworms. Parasites can cause harm to the host, and thus appropriate examinations should take place. While fleas, ticks, and lice are usually easily seen and identified, mites are too small, and thus require microscopic examination.

Scraping the skin for external parasite identification requires a number 10 scalpel, mineral oil in a dropper bottle, microscope slides, and a microscope. The scalpel blade is first moistened on a slide laden with mineral oil. It is then ready to obtain a scraping. The blade of the scalpel should be held in a perpendicular position towards the skin to ensure that an incision in the skin is not accidentally made. Grasp the skin gently between the thumb and index finger of one hand. The other hand should be used to make contact with the skin as the scraping motion is performed. Some parasites require deeper scrapes than other parasites. Therefore, a tentative determination should be made to classify the presenting case according to potential types: sarcoptes (burrowing mites), Demodex (hair follicle mites), Chorioptes, and Cheyletiella (both surface, non-burrowing skin mites). The burrowing mites require a deep scrape or rub to be collected.

Identification of burrowing external parasitic mites

Non-burrowing mites such as Demodex, Chorioptes, and Cheyletiella require only superficial skin scraping or rubbing for specimen collection. This should be sufficient to dislodge the loose scales and skin crusts in which they live. Scales are flaky pieces of skin. Crusts are dry, hardened outer layers of blood, pus, or other bodily secretion that forms over a cut or sore on the skin. Cheyletiella is sometimes referred to as "walking dandruff" due to the mites' habit of carrying dermal scales (i.e., dandruff) over the surface of the host. Burrowing mites (Sarcoptes) are more difficult to collect. To ensure adequate material collection, the skin in an affected area should be taken down just deep enough to produce a slow leak of blood. The material that is collected through either scraping method should be placed on a prepared slide laden with mineral oil. The slide should then be covered with a coverslip. The slide is scrutinized under a microscope at 10 power magnification. At least 10 slides should be inspected to ensure accuracy in making the external parasite identification.

Baermann Technique

There are 4 categories of endoparasites, often classified according to the part of the body they infect: blood, digestive system, organs, and sinus cavities. Many parasites have a life cycle that results in the presence of eggs (oocytes), larva, or the parasites themselves in excreted feces. The Baermann Technique is one test used to examine fecal matter for parasites and parasitic ova and larva. One of the parasites found in the feces is lungworm, living in the larval stage. The lungworm is a form of roundworm that lives in the pulmonary tissues of mammals and birds. Lungworm is introduced into the body through the ingestion of a contaminated food source. This worm can cause the host to have a number of respiratory problems. One indication of lungworm infestation is a severe cough.

The external identification of this parasite is accomplished via the Baermann Technique. It requires the use of a paper cup, disposable cellulose tissue or Kimwipe, elastic band, sedimentation jar, long Pasteur pipette with a bulb, and a dissecting microscope. A small amount of feces is examined for the presence of the lungworm. The feces sample is collected in the paper cup. A Kimwipe or a disposable cellulose tissue is placed on the cup as a cover. This cover is held in place with an elastic band.

The Baermann Technique for fecal examination requires a small hole to be made in the underside of the cup containing a fecal specimen. The cup must be covered with a Kimwipe or disposable cellulose tissue, which is secured with an elastic band. Warm water is used to fill a sedimentation jar halfway. Then, the cup should be submerged with the Kimwipe or cellulose tissue-end placed facedown in the water. All of the tissue should be in the water. The sample requires submersion in this manner for 12 to 18 hours.

After ample time has elapsed, a sample of water should be collected from the underside of the sedimentation jar. The sample is collected using a long Pasteur pipette with bulb. This is a small glass tube that allows liquid to be drawn into it by use of an attached suction bulb. At least 3 or 4 samples should be collected. The samples should be inspected under a dissecting microscope. The examination should show movement by any living larvae. Diligent perusal of the feces sample should allow ample opportunity for the external parasite to be identified. Lungworm can produce death in the host animal, and thus prompt treatment is essential.

Direct smear method

Fecal matter may also be examined for parasitic infestation by way of a glass slide smear. The direct smear method is also used to discover the existence of protozoa in feces. Protozoa are single cell organisms that feed on organic compounds. The direct smear method can aid in a rough calculation of the number of parasites present within the body. The direct smear method requires the following: microscope slides, coverslips, and applicator sticks. Lugol's iodine or methylene blue stain may be used, but neither is required. Fresh fecal matter is also required (at or near body temperature and ideally less than an hour old). Trophozoites in older specimens will lose motility, degenerate, and become very difficult if not impossible to recognize.

A single drop of saline solution (not water, which may rupture trophozoites) should be placed alongside an equal amount of feces on the surface of the slide. If stain is to be applied, then it should be added at this juncture. The blending of the feces and saline solution is accomplished with an applicator stick. This blend is thinly spread across the flat surface of the glass plate or slide. The larger pieces of feces are removed for uniform magnification and ease in slide viewing. Parasite eggs can be viewed with a 10-power magnification objective. Protozoal organisms can be viewed using a 40-power magnification objective.

Standard vial gravitation flotation technique

The standard vial gravitation flotation technique is used to find parasitic eggs in fecal matter. The principles and processes involved are not difficult. Further, the cost of this test is fairly low, which is an added benefit. However, this test may also be inaccurate, with false negative results not uncommon. The accuracy can be jeopardized by numerous variables in the testing process. The primary variable is the relative specific gravity of the flotation solution chosen. With the density of water as the reference point, a solution of higher specific gravity should cause parasite eggs or oocytes to float to the surface as the eggs have a lower specific gravity than the floating solution. However, different parasites have oocysts of varying specific gravity, and thus flotation may not always occur. Further, old fecal samples may experience egg degradation and altered flotation patterns, and poor straining strategies may trap eggs and remove them from the flotation solution.

The standard vial gravitation technique requires a paper cup filled with about 60 mL of floating solution. Then, 2 to 4 grams of feces is placed into the solution. The feces are handled with a tongue depressor. The solution and the feces are blended thoroughly. The blended solution is filtered through a strainer and poured into a second cup. This results in the reduction of extraneous waste material. This strained or filtered mixture is gently churned to disperse the eggs.

The final stages of the standard vial gravitation flotation technique require that this churned mixture be poured into a glass vial. The vial is filled to the top until a positive meniscus (upward curving solution surface) is formed. A coverslip or cover glass is positioned on top of the vial at this juncture, making contact with the meniscus. Then, the eggs are permitted to float to the surface of the vial. The parasite eggs or oocysts should float since they have a lower specific gravity than the flotation solution.

Once this has been accomplished, the cover glass can be removed. The cover glass should be carefully lifted off in a straight, upward direction. The cover glass is placed on top of the glass slide. The slide is now ready to be systematically and painstakingly examined. A cautious inspection should reveal the parasite oocysts present in the waste material, and allow for proper parasite identification.

OVC Puddle Technique

The OVC Puddle Technique is utilized to detect and monitor Cryptosporidium oocysts or eggs in feces. This technique requires the use of a microscope, glass slide, and coverslip; applicator stick; and a saturated sugar solution, such as corn syrup. A very small measure of feces is blended with a bit of the sugar solution. This blended solution is placed on a slide. The cover glass is placed on the slide at this juncture. The sample should be examined under a microscope using a 40-power objective. The coloration of the Cryptosporidium Oocysts is a light pinkish color. These oocysts are not to be confused with fungal spores that can also be present in the waste material. Fungal spores can be similar in shape and size as the oocysts or eggs. However, the fungal spores will start to bud after a period of time has elapsed, while the eggs will not.

Buffy coat method

The buffy coat method is used to examine a blood specimen for blood parasites. When blood is placed in a centrifuge and spun at a high rate, the 3 primary components of blood are separated from each other. The top layer is clear plasma; the bottom layer is red blood cells. In between is the "buffy coat" – a thin, creamy-yellowish (sometimes greenish) layer of white blood cells. If the buffy coat is placed on glass slides and examined under a microscope, the presence of parasites in the blood can often be revealed. The method requires the following: microhematocrit tubes and sealer, centrifuge, microscope slides and coverslips, saline solution, methylene blue stain, and a small file or glass cutter.

A microhematocrit tube is filled with blood. This tube of blood goes through centrifuge process for 3 minutes. The packed cell volume (PCV) is then read (it is an important overall indicator of hematological health). Next, the tube is scored at the level of the buffy coat. Then the tube is cautiously snapped before lightly tapping the buffy coat onto a slide. The buffy coat layer is inspected under a microscope. One drop of saline solution and one drop of methylene blue stain are placed on the slide. A coverslip is then positioned over the sample. The slide is then inspected for the presence of microfilariae. Finally, the plasma is retrieved from the microhematocrit tube's residue to be evaluated for total protein. Total protein is a good indicator of overall animal health.

ELISA parasite antibody test

Parasitic blood infestations will cause the body to develop antibodies to the presence of these foreign bodies. The enzyme-linked immunosorbent assay (ELISA) kits detect these antigens in the blood. While this test can reveal a host's antibody response to parasites, it cannot detect the microfilariae themselves. ELISA tests are particularly beneficial in the detection of occult heartworm (Dirofilaria immitis). Commercial kits available for this use include Dirochek from Synbiotics, PetChek/Snap from Idexx, and Witness from Binax. The tests are performed on a tray with an indented surface. The kit supplies a membrane or wand that has parasite-specific monoclonal antibodies bound to its surface. Blood samples containing this particular antigen can thus become bound to the antibody. Next, an additional antibody is labeled with an enzyme and applied to the sample. This will also bind to the antigen. A color-producing agent is then applied.

If parasite-specific antibodies are present after the introduction of this agent, then an antibody-enzyme complex will be formed, producing a specific color. The specific color is an indicator that the antigen (i.e., the parasite) is present. If there is no parasite-specific antigen in the sample, the enzyme-labeled antibody will wash away without any color-change result.

Skin digestion technique

The skin digestion technique is useful for the identification of external parasites. Skin scraping samples which have a significant amount of scurf (scales, epidermal shards) and skin debris is ideal for the skin digestion technique. The following is required for this technique: 15 mL conical centrifuge tube, 4% NaOH solution, hot plate, beaker, and centrifuge. The scalpel is used to place the sample in the centrifuge tube. Then, about 10 mL of NaOH solution is applied to the sample within the centrifuge tube. Next, the tube is positioned in a glass beaker water bath and boiled for 5 to 10 minutes. The centrifuge tube is then placed in the centrifuge for 5 minutes at 1000 rpm. Upon removal of the tube, the supernatant should be poured off from the top of the tube. Then, a drop of the sediment should be placed on a microscope slide and covered with a coverslip. Finally, the slide should be inspected for parasites using a microscope which has been set at a 10-power objective.

Cellophane tape method

The cellophane tape method is beneficial in the identification of intestinal pinworms and skin mites. Pinworms are threadlike nematode worms that invade the intestines. Parasitic pinworms can be found in and around the perianal area, while mites can be found on the hair and on the surface of the skin. The cellophane tape method requires the following: cellophane tape, mineral oil, and a microscope slide. The cellophane tape method involves applying tape to the outside of the skin. The tape is used to pull off the outer epidermis and related debris from the skin's surface. This sample is left on the tape. Then, a single drop of mineral oil is applied to the surface of a glass microscope slide. The tape is then positioned on top of the oil on the microscope slide. Finally, the sample is examined closely under a microscope set at a

10-power objective. In this way it can be determined if there are pinworms or mites on the sample.

Dirofilaria immitis

The presence of Dirofilaria immitis, or heartworm, is evident in a variety of symptoms exhibited by the host. This parasite takes up residence within the heart and pulmonary artery of the host animal. Heartworms can infect dogs, cats, and other non-domestic animals. Most animals become infected through a mosquito bite. Another method of transmission is through a transplacental infection of microfilaria. The prepatent period is described as the time between the initial infection and the maturation of the parasite into an adult (typically, when the parasite begins laying eggs). From infection to maturation requires a period of 6 to 8 months.

Animals that have been infected by heartworm will exhibit symptoms of lethargy, exercise intolerance, and cough. The cough can be more noticeable when the animal is exercising. Animals that have had heartworms for a lengthy period may exhibit additional problematic symptoms. These symptoms include: severe weight loss, fainting, coughing up blood, and congestive heart failure. Animals that are more active can exhibit symptoms of heartworm infection earlier than those less active. Likewise, animals that are heavily infected may also exhibit earlier symptoms of heartworm infection. Preventive medicine can reduce the likelihood of infection by heartworm. In particular, animals should receive limited exposure to mosquito bites.

Toxocara cati

The Toxocara cati or feline roundworm may sometimes be visible in the vomit of an animal. Toxocara cati roundworms inhabit the small intestines. It takes about 8 weeks from initial infection until this parasite can be detected through clinical means. The fecal flotation method can be used to expose the dark brown, thick-walled, pitted eggs of Toxocara cati. However, the eggs are not always present in the feces. Therefore, it is entirely possible that the results of a fecal flotation test will produce a false negative result.

The Toxocara cati has a complex life cycle. Infection occurs through eating an infected host (rodents, beetles, earthworms), through ingesting infected maternal milk, or by direct ingestion of eggs (via vomitus, fecal matter, etc). The ingested eggs hatch inside the cat. After emerging from their eggs, the larvae enter the small intestines of the host animal. From this juncture, the larvae enter the circulatory system of the feline, and then migrate to the pulmonary system, where they are coughed up and swallowed into the stomach. There, the larvae mature and reproduce more eggs to be discharged from the body in the feces.

Mature Toxocara cati roundworms produce eggs. These eggs are discharged or expelled from the body in the fecal waste released by the feline. The development period outside of the body lasts for about 10 to 14 days, at which point the eggs are actively infective. An unsuspecting feline will become infected by eating the infective eggs, usually in another food product that is consumed by the animal. The process then has begun all over again in this new unsuspecting host.

Kittens can be infected by drinking the infected milk of a mother cat. The infected cat's vomit will often have visible signs of the worms. The recommended treatment for roundworm or toxocara cati is the use of an appropriate medical deworming agent. Laboratory and physical symptoms of Toxocara cati include: 1) for visceral (intestinal) larva migrans – hypereosinophilia, hepatosplenomegaly, pneumonitis, fever, and hyperglobulinemia; and 2) ocular (eye) larva migrans (endophthalmitis) – leukokoria, loss of vision in the affected eye, eye pain, and strabismus. Cats are the primary host, but humans can become infected.

Dipylidium caninum

The diagnostic characteristics of Dipylidium caninum tapeworm can be seen in both dogs and cats. The prepatent period for Dipylidium caninum (the time between the initial infection and reproductive maturation) is about 3 weeks. This form of tapeworm resides in the small intestines of infected dogs and cats. The tapeworm itself presents with a long ribbon-shaped body. These worms have a head, neck, and segmented body parts. The segmented body parts are formed unceasingly in the neck region of the worm. The older segments are found on the tip of the worm's body. These older segments (gravid proglottids) are discarded at maturational intervals. The discarded proglottid segments are able to independently reproduce, as each contains both male and female reproductive organs. The segments stay active as long as host warmth is retained. Finally, the segment opens up in order to release the eggs that are inside. These eggs are eaten by an adult louse or flea larva, ultimately to infect or be ingested by another animal.

Flea or louse larvae may ingest the eggs of Dipylidium caninum, whereupon the insect becomes infected. The potential cat or dog that ingests the adult louse or flea will become infected. This tapeworm parasite is able to grow into adulthood inside the animal's body. Eventually the animal discharges fecal matter that contains gravid (egg-bearing) tapeworm segments known as proglottids. These proglottids have a complete reproductive system. A clinical inspection, in the form of a fecal flotation examination, can expose proglottid segments.

The animal that has this type of infestation may be seen scrubbing its bottom across the surface of the ground. The animal may find this scrubbing action brings relief to itching and irritation in the area around the anus. This discomfort may be caused by active segments of the parasite found near the anus. Sometimes, detection can be made through inspection of the feces for more obvious segments of the tapeworm. The infected animal should be treated with medications. However, a preventive stance is recommended — principally to reduce the animal's exposure to fleas or lice infestations.

Ancylostoma caninum

Ancylostoma caninum (or "dog hookworm") is defined as a hookworm that takes up residence in the small intestines of canines. Hookworms are blood-sucking parasites that can cause significant disease in the host animal. The hookworm fastens itself to the wall of the small intestine. There, the hookworm proceeds to feed on the animal's blood. Feeding is accomplished via intestinal wall penetration using its hook-like mouth. In most cases, infection occurs when an adult dog ingests the eggs or larvae by consuming food or water that has been contaminated. The soil around the animal may also become contaminated with the larvae of the hookworm. Another method of infection occurs when a dog consumes an infected host. The canine may also become infected by larval penetration through the animal's skin. Further, young canine pups may become infected through mammary glands by drinking its mother's milk. Finally, the fetus may be infected through the uterus via the placenta. The parasite can be detected 2 to 3 weeks after the initial infection.

The dog hookworm parasite (Ancylostoma caninum) can be detected by fecal flotation testing. The parasite's eggs can be observed as clear, smooth, thin-walled eggs found in the feces. The worms are not usually seen by the naked eye due to their small size. The worms range in size from about ½ to ¾ inches in length. Further, the hookworm is capable of fastening itself firmly to the wall or lining of the small intestine, and thus is not normally dislodged. Ancylostoma caninum can have very detrimental effects on the host animal. Some of the more severe symptoms include anemia, weakness, and melena. Anemia is a condition in which the blood is deficient. Melena is a condition in which the body produces black, tarry, blood-bearing feces. The blackened, tarry feces indicate that there is bleeding in the bowel region (rather than up higher, where it would have been all or at least partially digested). This parasite infection can be treated with proper medical care. However, a preventive stance is recommended, reducing the animal's exposure to feces within its immediate surroundings.

Trichuris vulpis

Trichuris vulpis, or Whipworm, is a type of nematode or roundworm that can be found in human and canine intestines. The whipworm gets its name from its shape, similar to a whip. The whipworm resides in the cecum and large intestines of canines. The prepatent period (from infestation to maturation) is about 3 months. An animal is infected by whipworm through the consumption of food or drink that has been contaminated with infective eggs. In the process of digestion, the eggs hatch, and migrate into the cecum where they grow into larvae and then develop into adulthood. This development process within the cecum (which marks the start of the large intestines) takes a period of 3 months. The whipworm migrates out of the cecum and into the large intestine of the animal. There, the whipworm attaches itself to the intestinal wall. Once attached, the whipworm finds nourishment from blood drawn through the intestinal wall and capillary penetration.

The Trichuris vulpis worm is detected by viewing the eggs in the feces. This viewing is accomplished through the fecal flotation technique. The animal may experience a range of symptoms depending upon the amount of worms present in the animal. A small number of worms may not produce any observable symptoms. Animals with a large infection of worms may have more severe symptoms. Symptoms include: extreme and severe watery diarrhea, bright red blood in the stool, rapid dehydration, and even death.

The immature larvae may be resistant to certain medical interventions. However, most medications are effective in the treatment of adult whipworms. The animal can be expected to need medical treatment for a period of several months. This allows all the larvae to mature so that they can be effectively eradicated in adulthood. Preventive care is recommended, and involves the removal of feces from the animal's surrounding area. The fecal matter can increase risk of infection as it may have active eggs that have been excreted from an infected animal's body.

Isospora ssp

Isospora ssp (subspecies) is one of many sporozoan intestinal parasites of the order Coccidia. As a Coccidian, it is a spore-forming single-celled (protozoan) parasite. This parasite infects both cats and dogs. Coccidia parasites typically take up residence in the small intestines of an animal. Diseases that occur as a result of these protozoa fall under the descriptive header of coccidiosis. Puppies and kittens that range in age from birth to 6 months of age are susceptible to the disease. Adult animals that have a suppressed immune system can also be susceptible to this disease. Stress can cause the immune system to be weakened to a point that the animal finds itself more susceptible to this infection. The prepatent period, the time of infestation to maturation, can range from 4 to 12 days. Puppies or kittens are usually around the age of 2 weeks or more when they contract coccidiosis. This disease can be detected by the fecal flotation method.

The canine or feline with Isospora ssp (subspecies) coccidiosis has been infected by the consumption of the parasite's eggs. The most prominent symptoms are frequent and excessive bowel movements consisting of soft, fluid-laden diarrhea. The severity of the diarrhea may be indicative of the acuteness of the infection. Because of the copious fluids expelled in an effort to flush the parasites out, the animal experiencing acute symptoms may be in danger of dehydration and death.

The fecal material contains active eggs or oocysts that have been excreted with the feces from the infected animal's body. Upon proper examination, it will be noted that the infected stool contains many clear, spherical to ellipsoid, thin-walled oocysts that can best be detected by the fecal floatation method. Once coccidiosis is confirmed, the disease should be properly treated with medications and appropriate follow-up medical care. Preventive care is also highly recommended, and involves the removal of feces from the animal's surrounding area, as the continuing presence of infected fecal matter can increase risk of recurrent infection.

Giardia duodenalis

Giardia duodenalis, or simply "Giardia," is a single-cell protozoan that can intestinally infect an animal. Infection occurs when the host ingests dormant cysts found in contaminated water, or by consuming food contaminated with moist feces that host the parasite. As the cysts can survive for months in a moist environment – even in cold, clean-appearing water, including water treated for city drinking – infections are difficult to avoid. Once ingested, the Giardia parasite fastens itself to the surface of an animal's small intestines. These protozoans may also be found moving freely along the mucosal lining of an animal's intestines.

Giardia can infect a number of mammals, including dogs, cats, cattle, horses, sheep, goats, and pigs. Infected animals develop severe symptoms of diarrhea. Giardia duodenalis has 2 basic life cycle states: trophozoite and cystic. In the metabolically active (feeding) stage the Giardia protozoa are known as trophozoites. Possessing a flagellum, the trophozoite is motile – meaning it can move freely as it seeks nourishment. The other life cycle state is the non-motile cystic stage. At the conclusion of the trophozoite life stage, the protozoa rapidly replicate via binary fission, and then transform themselves into inactive cysts. Upon expulsion from the host, the cysts quickly become infective and thrive in any moist environment for several months.

The cycle of Giardia duodenalis infection continues when a new host is attacked. The new host typically consumes water or food that has been contaminated with Giardia cysts. The infection spreads rapidly, as the infective cysts break open in the intestines of the new host animal. These broken cysts release the now metabolically active trophozoite into the new host animal. The prepatent period, the time period from initial infestation to reproductive maturity, for Giardia is 7 to 10 days.

The fecal flotation method is usually effective in making a diagnosis of the infection. Another method used is the direct smear technique. A diagnosis is confirmed when either the cysts or the trophozoites are viewed. The cysts present a smooth, thin-walled protective covering which protects the parasite held inside. The trophozoite has a piriform (pear or teardrop) shape. The trophozoite has bilateral symmetry and a light coloration of green. Giardia can be effectively treated with medication and proper follow-up medical care.

Cheyletiella spp

Cheyletiella (the name used by acarologists – those who study mites and ticks) has long been called "walking dandruff" for the mite's propensity to carry skin scales around with them as they move about. Cheyletiella mites can infest dogs, cats, and rabbits. Mites are creatures with 8 legs that extend beyond the margins of their bodies. The adult mite is oval in shape, and can take up residence on the host's skin surface or on hair shafts or in hair follicles. The mite's stages of development require approximately 21-35 days for completion. The entire life cycle takes place on the host.

The adult mite is capable of living for 2-14 days off the body of the host. When off the host, mites have the ability to infect an animal through environmental contacts. Even so, mites normally infect an animal through more direct contact (i.e., moving among animals that come into physical contact with each other). Walking dandruff has the following symptoms: obvious scurf or dandruff scales, visible mites on the surface of the skin, pruritus (itching, resulting in scratching for relief), inflammation of the skin, crusts, and small swellings or spots. Walking dandruff is detected by skin scrapings, the cellophane tape method, combings, or via microscopic study. Once diagnosed, walking dandruff can be treated with appropriate medications.

Ctenocephalides spp

There are 2 common species of Ctenocephalides spp (subspecies). A widely found species is the cat flea known to pulicologists (those who study fleas) as Ctenocephalides felis. Another species is the dog flea, which is known as Ctenocephalides canis. While the dog flea is rarely found, the cat flea is routinely found on both cats and dogs. An animal that has been infected by the cat flea may be diagnosed through readily visible evidence. Adult fleas take up residence and grow on the host's skin. Adult fleas lay eggs, which fall off the host in areas that the host frequents (bedding, living areas, etc).

Upon hatching (in 1-6 days) the larvae exist on organic debris and adult flea feces (requisite to their continued development). The larvae range in size from about 1.5 to 5 mm in length. Upon larval maturation they spin a cocoon in which they reside as a "pupa" – an insect in a metamorphosis stage. After 1-2 weeks the pupa is a fully developed adult flea. However, the pupa will not leave the cocoon until adequate environmental stimuli indicate they are near a suitable host (e.g., heat, physical pressure, carbon dioxide, or movement). If no stimulus prompts emergence, the flea can remain in a quiescent cocoon state for up to 350 days.

Adult flea coloration is reddish-brown to black in appearance. The adults do not have wings, but are able to jump great distances. The adults have a life span that ranges from about 4-25 days in length, receiving nourishment by biting and drinking the blood of the host. The flea is a parasitic insect which can rapidly spread by leaping onto other hosts and surfaces. The animal that has been infected by fleas may experience flea allergy dermatitis (as may humans who sometimes briefly become secondary hosts).

Dermatitis is an inflammation that appears as redness, itching, and/or swelling of the skin. Animals with this condition may exhibit symptoms such as scratching excessively. This scratching can further damage the animal's skin. The animal should be closely observed in order to detect fleas or residual flea feces. Flea feces appear as small specks of dirt on the animal. Where discovered, treatment should take place. The bedding and living environment of the animal should also be checked and treated, if necessary. Preventive care is recommended to reduce exposure to the infection.

Lice

There are 2 kinds of lice. The sucking lice are called Anoplura. The biting lice are called Mallophaga. Different species of Anoplura attack different species of animals. The species known as Haematopinus spp will infect cattle, pigs, and horses. The species known as Linognathus spp infects dogs, cattle, and sheep. The species known as Solenopotes spp infects cattle. The species known as Pediculus spp infects humans. Likewise, different species of

Mallophaga attack different species of animals. The species known as Damalinia spp (subspecies) infects horses, cattle, and sheep. The species known as Felicola subrostratus infects felines. The species known as Trichodectes canis infects dogs. These 2 different kinds of lice have certain commonalities. For example, the adult lice have similar shapes — dorsoventrally flattened with the head narrower than the thorax. "Dorsoventral" refers to the belly-to-back anatomical axis.

Those animals that become infected may have lice on their skin and in their hair. Lice lay eggs, which are known as nits. The nits are typically glued to the hair shaft so as not to fall from the host. Lice are also transferred from one host to another through physical contact. Lice have the ability to spend an entire life cycle on a single animal or host. Lice infestation is typically readily evident through close observation. The parasites are visible on inspection. Further, the animal may exhibit excessive itchiness, accompanied by a scruffy, dry, or brittle hair or fur coat.

When infestation is evident, the animal or human should be deloused. Delousing will free the person of lice through the application of a medication. This treatment is designed to kill the lice. Preventive care is highly recommended. Medication should be applied to all the surfaces with which the animal has had contact. This includes the animal's bedding and surrounding living area. Failure to fully treat the animal and all the infective surfaces can readily result in a reinfestation of the lice. Reinfestation will likely require yet another thorough treatment to be applied to the animal and all surfaces involved.

Strongylus vulgaris

Strongylus vulgaris is an equine intestinal worm ranging in length up to 25 mm. This worm takes up residence in the large intestine of a horse. The prepatent period of the equine worm can range from about 6-12 months in duration. Non-infective eggs are discharged in the feces when a host animal defecates. Following excretion, the eggs go through a developmental process in stages. The eggs move from first stage larvae, or the L1 stage, to the second or L2 stage without becoming infective. This is followed by the third or L3 stage. It is in this last stage of development that the larvae become infective. After the L3 stage and upon ingestion, the larva sheds its protective sheath or covering (called "ex-sheathing"). This allows the larvae to migrate and eventually to pierce the walls of the intestines at or below the cecum. The cecum is the first intestinal pouch, at the point of which the large intestine originates.

Once the Strongylus vulgaris larva has penetrated the intestinal wall, it travels further until it enters the submucosa. The submucosa is the layer of connective tissue directly beneath the mucus membrane of the intestine. Horses that have been infected by the equine worm will experience a range of clinical signs. The signs of infection include colic, fever, diarrhea, weight loss, and death. Colic is a pain that occurs in the abdominal region, typically due to spasm, obstruction or distention of the viscera.

A Strongylus vulgaris infection can be detected via the fecal flotation method. The larvae in stages 1 and 2 can be killed easily. At these stages the larvae exist largely in residual manure.

Thus, the spreading and breaking up of manure is an effective deterrent to the growth and development of the larva. There is also treatment available for larvae that reach stage 3 and then become adult worms. Treatment can be found in the form of antiparasitic medications that can be administered to the horse.

Practice Test

Multiple Choice Questions

1. Rattlesnake envenomation produces this type of poikilocyte: B
   a. Spherocytes
   b. Echinocytes
   c. Acanthocytes
   d. Schistocytes

2. Over-the-counter nonsteroidal anti-inflammatory drugs (NSAIDs) such as ibuprofen, naproxen, and aspirin represent a leading cause of toxicoses in small animals. What is their common mechanism of action?
   a. Bone marrow suppression
   b. Smooth muscle contraction
   c. Prostaglandin synthesis inhibition
   d. Vasodilation of renal vessels

3. Improper handling or restraint of rabbits can result in this common injury: B
   a. Diaphragmatic hernia
   b. Spinal fracture or luxation
   c. Splenic rupture
   d. Skull fracture

4. Which small mammal has a high risk of dystocia if bred after 6 months of age?   C
   a. Chinchilla
   b. Rabbit
   c. Guinea pig
   d. Ferret

5. Animals poisoned with ethylene glycol (antifreeze) often have large numbers of these crystals in the urine:
   a. Struvite
   b. Ammonium biurate
   c. Cystine
   d. Calcium oxalate

6. Which of the following statements regarding dermatophyte test medium (DTM) is TRUE?
   a. Sample DTM jars should be closed tightly to prevent the introduction of saprophytic fungi.
   b. Dermatophytes rapidly change the color of the DTM agar to red in as little as 3-5 days.
   c. Samples should be placed in an incubator for 1-2 weeks.
   d. All of the above.

7. In a nonrebreathing system, which of the following has the most influence on the amount of carbon dioxide (CO_2) rebreathed?
   a. Fresh gas flow rate
   b. CO2 absorbent
   c. Scavenger system
   d. Design of rebreathing system

8. What will happen to a patient if the positive-pressure-relief (pop-off) valve is accidentally left closed during anesthesia?
   a. Pressure will build up in the system and the patient will not be able to exhale.
   b. The lungs will rupture causing a pneumothorax, a life-threatening emergency.
   c. Venous return to the heart will be compromised.
   d. All of the above.

9. An increase in heart rate that is accompanied with normal P-QRS-T complexes on electrocardiogram (ECG), and occurs as a result of increased activity of the sinoatrial (SA) node is termed:
   a. Ventricular tachycardia
   b. Atrial fibrillation
   c. Sinus tachycardia
   d. Atrial tachycardia

10. What drug is the emetic of choice in canines?
   a. Xylazine
   b. Apomorphine
   c. Hydrogen peroxide
   d. Syrup of ipecac

11. A technician is about to administer an intramuscular injection of antibiotic to a box turtle suffering from an aural abscess. Where should the technician administer this injection?
   a. Front leg
   b. Back leg
   c. None of the above
   d. a or b

12. Which of the following statements is NOT true regarding jugular intravenous drug administration in horses?
   a. The needle should be inserted caudally into the jugular vein in order to match the direction of blood flow.
   b. The cranial third of the neck should be used to access the jugular vein to avoid accidental entry into the carotid artery.
   c. The medication should be bolused as quickly as possible.
   d. Arterial versus venous blood cannot be differentiated by color when drawn into a syringe filled with fluid.

13. Which of the following syndromes will result in a postrenal azotemia?
   a. Shock
   b. Antifreeze intoxication
   c. Feline urologic syndrome (FUS).
   d. Dehydration

- 97 -

14. A 75-pound Labrador Retriever requires 8 mg/kg of injectable phenobarbital for initial treatment of status epilepticus. If the concentration of this drug is 30 mg/mL, how many milliliters should this patient receive?
    a. 9 mL
    b. 20 mL
    c. 60 mL
    d. 18 mL

15. Which of the following statements regarding grids is incorrect?
    a. Grids help reduce the amount of scatter radiation.
    b. Grids are used when the area to be radiographed is equal to or exceeds 10 cm in thickness.
    c. Grids do not absorb any part of the primary beam.
    d. Grids improve the quality of the radiograph by increasing contrast.

16. A client brings in his 5-month-old puppy for vomiting and diarrhea of 2-day duration. He indicates that he himself vaccinated the puppy with injectables purchased at a local feed and grain store. He also states that he followed a vaccine protocol described on the Internet. Despite this owner's good intentions, the puppy tests positive for parvovirus. What is a plausible explanation for this test result?
    a. The puppy was immunosuppressed at the time of vaccination and could therefore not mount a sufficient immune response to the vaccines.
    b. The owner administered the vaccine incorrectly or at inappropriate intervals.
    c. The vaccine was stored at an improper temperature by the retail store or by the owner, thereby rendering the vaccine ineffective.
    d. All of the above.

17. Which of the following statements regarding feline transfusion medicine is incorrect?
    a. There is no universal feline blood type due to the presence of naturally occurring alloantibodies.
    b. Type A cats have weak anti-B alloantibodies.
    c. A type AB cat can be safely used as an in-house blood donor.
    d. Transfusion of a type B cat with type A blood can produce a potentially fatal acute hemolytic crisis.

18. Alkaline urine does not result from, nor is produced by
    a. Diets rich in vegetable products.
    b. A urinary tract infection with urease producing bacteria (ie, Staph or Proteus).
    c. Time (>1 hr the voided sample stands at room temperature).
    d. Diets consisting of milk or animal products.

19. What type of drug is activated charcoal?
    a. Laxative
    b. Cathartic
    c. Purgative
    d. Adsorbent and protectant

20. Which of the following is NOT a function of diazepam?
    a. Anxiolytic
    b. Anticonvulsant
    c. Analgesic
    d. Muscle relaxant

- 98 -

21. What is the earliest day of gestation that a small animal pregnancy can be confirmed using ultrasound?
    a. Day 5
    b. Day 11
    c. Day 20
    d. Day 45

22. The components of fresh whole blood remain effective for up to:
    a. 1 hour
    b. 2 hours
    c. 8 hours
    d. 12 hours

23. What type of injection should be avoided in meat-producing animals?
    a. Subcutaneous
    b. Intravenous
    c. Intramuscular
    d. Intraperitoneal

24. What is ultimately responsible for the resolution of an ultrasound image?
    a. Size of patient
    b. Gain
    c. Transducer frequency
    d. Power

25. On electrocardiograms (ECGs), ectopic foci that discharge prematurely anywhere within the ventricular walls give rise to:
    a. Ventricular tachycardia
    b. Ventricular fibrillation
    c. Ventricular premature complexes
    d. Accelerated idioventricular rhythm

26. What is the most commonly encountered diet-related illness in pet hedgehogs?
    a. Rickets
    b. Obesity
    c. Hepatic lipidosis
    d. Periodontal disease

27. In ultrasonography, this artifact is produced when soundwaves are unable to traverse certain types of tissue or anomalies, such as bone or calculi:
    a. Distance enhancement
    b. Reverberation
    c. Acoustic shadowing
    d. Mirror image

28. What is the anesthetic of choice in patients with cardiac disease?
    a. Ketamine
    b. Propofol
    c. Fentanyl
    d. Etomidate

29. Etomidate should not be administered in repeated boluses because it is a hypertonic solution. What term best describes the changes a red blood cell (RBC) undergoes when introduced into a hypertonic solution?
    a. Autoagglutination
    b. Hemolysis
    c. Crenation
    d. Rouleaux formation

30. Which of the following statements regarding equine nasogastric intubation and medication is FALSE?
    a. The nasogastric tube should be guided into the dorsal meatus of the horse's nasal passages.
    b. When placed properly, the tube can be seen on the left side of the horse's neck as it passes through the esophagus and into the stomach.
    c. Force should NEVER be used at any time during nasogastric intubation.
    d. A horse could potentially die from gastric rupture when its stomach is overfilled with large volumes of medication or fluid delivered through a nasogastric tube

31. Which of the following statements regarding urine casts is TRUE?
    a. Large numbers of casts in urine usually indicate active renal disease.
    b. Casts will dissolve in alkaline urine.
    c. Casts contain material in their matrix that was present in the renal tubule when the cast was formed.
    d. All of the above.

32. Which of the following is the most common oropharyngeal tumor in canines?
    a. Fibrosarcoma
    b. Squamous cell carcinoma
    c. Malignant melanoma
    d. Ameloblastoma

33. Cutaneous larval migrans is an important parasitic zoonoses that is caused by:
    a. Whipworms
    b. Roundworms
    c. Tapeworms
    d. Hookworms

34. The connective tissue that occupies the space between each tooth and the alveolar bone is called:
    a. Cementum
    b. Pulp
    c. Periodontal ligament
    d. Gingiva

35. What is the purpose of polishing in dental prophylaxis?
    a. Eliminate calculi
    b. Remove sublingual deposits
    c. Strengthen the enamel
    d. Smooth the enamel

36. Mechanical scalers have the potential to generate excessive heat on the enamel, which can lead to accidental structural damage to the tooth. What step(s) can be taken to avoid this scenario?
    a. Use a large amount of water to cool the teeth during scaling.
    b. Limit the time spent on each tooth to 5-10 seconds each.
    c. Use only at the recommended speed for the particular unit.
    d. All of the above.

37. Scissors that are primarily used in intraocular surgery are called:
    a. Metzenbaum scissors
    b. Iris scissors
    c. Mayo scissors
    d. Spencer scissors

38. Large hemostatic forceps with longitudinal grooves along the opposing blade surfaces and transverse grooves at the tip are called:
    a. Kelly forceps
    b. Rochester-Carmalt forceps
    c. Mosquito forceps
    d. Crile forceps

39. What is the function of surgical milk on instruments?
    a. Lubrication
    b. Sterilization
    c. Anti-corrosive
    d. Both a and c

40. In a rebreathing system, how often should the carbon dioxide absorbent be changed?
    a. Every 2-4 hours of use
    b. Every 6-8 hours of use
    c. Every 10-12 hours of use
    d. Every 20 hours of use

41. Which knot is recommended to secure a patient's limb to the surgery table?
    a. Square knot
    b. Sheet bend knot
    c. Bowline knot
    d. Half hitch

42. Drain placement helps to reduce the occurrence of
    a. Seromas.
    b. Dead space.
    c. Hematomas.
    d. All of the above.

43. Which of the following statements regarding hydrogen peroxide (H_2O_2) is FALSE?
    a. Hydrogen peroxide is an effective broad spectrum antimicrobial.
    b. Hydrogen peroxide can damage tissue with repeated use.
    c. Hydrogen peroxide is a common foaming wound irrigant.
    d. Hydrogen is an effective sporicide.

44. Which of the following properties is NOT shared by chlorhexidine AND povidone-iodine scrubs?
    a. They are both broad-spectrum antimicrobials.
    b. Their residual bactericidal effects are inactivated by blood or alcohol.
    c. They have a rapid antimicrobial effect.
    d. They both have residual antimicrobial activity that lasts more than 3 hours.

45. Which of the following should never be used to maintain or increase the body temperature of an animal that is undergoing or recovering from surgery?
    a. Heated circulating water blanket
    b. Electric heating pad
    c. Warm water bath
    d. Warm air blanket

46. Which of the following pairs of analgesics should NOT be used together?
    a. Morphine and lidocaine
    b. Butorphanol and fentanyl
    c. Dexmedetomidine and buprenorphine
    d. Tramadol and nonsteroidal anti-inflammatory drugs

47. Which of the following opioids can be administered transmucosally in the feline?
    a. Buprenorphine
    b. Hydroxymorphone
    c. Fentanyl
    d. Butorphanol

48. Which of the following drugs is used to offset the untoward effect of hypersalivation that is commonly seen with barbiturate and dissociative anesthetics?
    a. Naloxone hydrochloride
    b. Antisedan
    c. Glycopyrrolate
    d. Thiopental

49. Stay sutures are used to
    a. Elevate and stabilize hollow organs.
    b. Separate muscle layers.
    c. Secure a chest tube to the skin.
    d. Prevent recurrence of a rectal prolapse.

50. All of the following drugs are diuretics EXCEPT:
    a. Furosemide.
    b. Enalapril.
    c. Spironolactone.
    d. Mannitol.

Multiple Choice Answers

1. B: Echinocytes are small, crenated (shrunken) erythrocytes characterized by the presence of 10-30 spikes or spicules on their outer membrane. Normally they are most numerous within the first 24 hours of envenomation, before the development of clinical signs, and will affect almost 100% of the red blood cells. After 2-3 days, the echinocytes steadily decrease in number and eventually become absent on a blood smear. It is important to note, however, that in some animals echinocytes do not appear at all following envenomation and that appropriate medical therapy will still need to be implemented.

2. C: Prostaglandins are chemicals that mediate an array of normal physiologic functions such as platelet aggregation, renal blood flow, and gastric acid production. In addition, they protect the cells lining the gastrointestinal (GI) tract from noxious chemicals. When over-the-counter NSAIDs are mistakenly given or accidentally ingested in large quantities, they work to inhibit prostaglandin synthesis, which can potentially lead to a myriad of life-threatening problems such as GI ulceration, clotting abnormalities, and kidney failure.
It is important to note that the toxic dose of any NSAID can vary between animals depending on individual sensitivities, and actual manifestation of clinical signs (melena, vomiting, etc) can be delayed by up to 4 days following ingestion. This being said, many owners do not seek out veterinary care unless clinical signs are present and only after the damage has already been done. Thus, it is important to recommend to clients who may have administered or suspect that their animals have ingested any NSAID that their animal be seen immediately for a consultation.

3. B: Rabbits that are allowed to frantically kick, whether confined in a cage or while being restrained, or rabbits that are dropped can fracture or dislocate their lumbar vertebrae. The result is hind limb paresis or paralysis that only rarely responds to emergency medical therapy.
When handled or restrained, rabbits need to have their hind end fully supported. This can be accomplished with a "football" hold, whereby the rabbit's head is tucked into the handler's arm with one hand, and the other hand supports its hind end. If rabbits are kept at the clinic and become too excited in a cage, then they will need to be moved to a small carrier to prevent excessive movement.

4. C: The pubic symphysis of guinea pigs fuses together between 7 and 8 months of age and is normally not an issue with nonbreeding females. Guinea pigs that are acquired for breeding purposes, however, and are bred after 6 months of age will experience difficult labor and possibly dystocia if they are unable to separate the symphysis during parturition.

5. D: Calcium oxalate monohydrate urolithiasis is a common occurrence in animals that have ingested antifreeze (ethylene glycol). It occurs as a result of ethylene glycol metabolism in the liver, the end products of which are several potentially lethal toxic metabolites, one of which is oxalate. These metabolites direct their toxic effects on the kidneys by destroying renal epithelial cells as well as by obstructing the renal tubules, which ultimately results in acute renal failure.

6. B: Dermatophytes can quickly change the color of the DTM agar to red in as few as 3-5 days, and before growth can be visualized by the naked eye. The caps on these samples need to be secured loosely to permit the flow of air into the sample, thus allowing growth of the dermatophyte. The sample should be kept at room temperature in a place where it can be easily seen and evaluated each day.

7. A: In a nonrebreathing system, there is no CO_2 absorption, so the clearance of CO_2 is dependent on the use of high fresh gas flow rates (200-300 mL/kg/min). These rates are required to prevent buildup of CO_2, which can lead to the rebreathing of exhaled air. Flow rates below 200 mL/kg/min will result in the accumulation and rebreathing of exhaled gases, and the potential for the development of hypoxemia and hypercarbemia.

8. D: A pop-off valve that is accidentally left closed during anesthesia can have catastrophic repercussions. Pressure will build up in the system, and as a result, the patient will not be able to exhale. If pressure continues to build in the thorax, there will be inadequate venous return to the heart. Ultimately, a patient could suffer a ruptured lung and subsequent pneumothorax. Thus, it is EXTREMELY important to remember to open a pop-off valve that has been closed, and always put the anesthetic machine away with the valve in the open position.

9. C: Sinus tachycardia is an increase in heart rate that can occur due to a variety of physiologic (ie, exercise, pain, fear), pharmacologic (drugs such as atropine, epinephrine, acepromazine) or pathologic influences (ie, anemia, heart failure, shock). The heart remains under the control of a normal SA node and the P-QRS-T complexes appear normal.

10. B: Apomorphine is the most reliable and effective drug for the induction of emesis in canines. When administered intravenously or intramuscularly, apomorphine can produce emesis in a matter of minutes. It is also available in a tablet form that can be crushed and a small amount placed in the conjunctival sac.
Xylazine is an effective and fast-acting (1-2 minutes) emetic in cats.
Hydrogen peroxide can induce vomiting in dogs by irritating the gastric mucosa. Results, however, are often not immediate and may not occur at all.
Syrup of ipecac can also induce vomiting in dogs, but only after 15-30 minutes following administration. It must reach the intestine before it exerts is effects.

11. A: The technician should administer the injection in a front leg in order to avoid the renal portal system in the caudal half of the body. The renal portal system is a complex of blood vessels associated with the kidneys. Injections given in the caudal half of the body could potentially be carried to the kidneys before entering the systemic circulation. As a result, the drug may not reach therapeutic levels because a portion may be excreted prematurely. Renal damage could also occur since the drug has not had an opportunity to be metabolized by the body.

12. C: Caution must always be exercised when performing an intravenous (IV) injection in the jugular vein of horses because the carotid artery lies in close proximity to the jugular vein, and can therefore be mistakenly accessed even by the most experienced technicians. Steps to help minimize this error include utilizing the cranial third of the neck for venipuncture. This is because the artery does not lie in such close proximity to the vein as it does in the more caudal aspect of the neck. Another tactic would be to insert a large bore needle first and watch the blood as it exits the hub. If it is a gentle drip, then the needle is in the vein. If it is a steady, pulsating stream, the needle is in the artery and needs to be readjusted. Once the needle is in the vein, the drug should be administered slowly in order to give the technician or veterinarian ample time to stop the injection in the event of an adverse reaction. For example, sometimes horses move during an injection and cause the needle to be redirected into the carotid artery. If medication is injected into the carotid artery, it travels straight to the brain where it can cause potentially lethal consequences. Thus, it is extremely important not to be overconfident with these injections, and always use good judgment and safe techniques.

Copyright © Mometrix Media. You have been licensed one copy of this document for personal use only.
Any other reproduction or redistribution is strictly prohibited. All rights reserved.

13. C: Postrenal azotemia results from either an obstruction (ie, foreign body, FUS, neoplasia) in the urinary outflow tract or interruption (ie, rupture, laceration) of the urinary outflow tract leading to the escape of urine into the peritoneal cavity. Early in the course of the disease, lab findings usually demonstrate an increase in both the blood urea nitrogen (BUN) and creatinine values. Urine specific gravity is usually normal. Postrenal azotemia, however, can progress to intrinsic renal disease due to increased pressure in the urinary system or due to a sustained decrease in renal blood flow. The prognosis of postrenal azotemia is good if the underlying cause can be treated or corrected early in the course of disease.

14. A: First, convert pounds to kilograms: 75 lbs * 1 kg/2.2 lbs = 34 kg. Second, calculate how many milligrams of drug the patient requires: 34 kg * 8 mg/kg = 272 mg. Third, calculate the volume that will yield 272 mg of drug: 272 mg * 1 mL/30 mg = 9 mL.

15. C: In radiology, grids are used to help reduce the amount of scatter radiation when radiographing large areas (≥10 cm thick). They are needed because larger subjects require more kVp for penetration, and more kVp produces more scatter radiation, which ultimately results in a poor quality radiograph. An important fact about grids is that they do indeed absorb some of the primary beam thereby necessitating an increase in exposure. This is accomplished by increasing the mAs before taking the radiograph.

16. D: The efficacy of any one vaccine is dependent on several variables. First and foremost, it must be stored in the proper conditions once it leaves the manufacturer. As a consumer, it is impossible to know if the store immediately refrigerated the vaccines after they arrived. Also, the consumer must transport the vaccine back home and may do so in less than optimal conditions. Perhaps this individual forgets that the vaccine is in the car, or runs errands on a hot day, thereby further endangering the vaccine's potency.
If the vaccine does happen to make it home without insult, there are still other variables that could produce a less than optimal immune response once it is injected. For example, the owner could inadvertently inject all the way through the skin, in which case the puppy receives no vaccine at all. If the owner starts the vaccine series too early (before 6 weeks), maternal antibodies will destroy the vaccine. Also, if the puppy is sick or is born with a weak immune system, it may not be able to mount a sufficient antibody response to the vaccine. In all these instances, vaccines will lose their efficacy, which is why it is important to educate the public about the dangers of store-bought vaccines and why exams are recommended before any vaccine is administered.

17. C: There are 3 described blood types in cats: A, B, and AB. Blood type A is the most prevalent and is seen in most domestic longhairs and shorthairs. Blood type B is not as common and is seen mostly in purebred cats, but not exclusively. Type AB is very rare and can be present in any cat. All cats have naturally occurring alloantibodies to blood types that are not their own. These antibodies can be very strong, as in the case of type B cats, or weak as with the type A cats. As a result, type B cats will undergo a severe reaction if transfused with type A blood. However, type A cats may not react at all with a transfusion of type B blood, but the transfused blood will only last a few days. Because of the presence of these alloantibodies, there can be no universal feline donor. A type AB cat is no exception.

18. D: Diets consisting of animal products and/or milk are acid producing and therefore, lower the pH of urine.

Diets rich in vegetable products will produce an alkaline urine sample.

A urine sample that is allowed to stand at room temperature for an hour or more will become alkaline, so these must be checked within 20-30 minutes of collection or at least refrigerated to help prevent the sample from degrading.

A urinary tract infection with urease producing bacteria will cause an alkaline urine sample because the enzyme urease converts urea to ammonia, which raises pH.

19. D: Activated charcoal adsorbs to its surface many chemicals, toxins, and drugs in the upper gastrointestinal tract that would otherwise be absorbed systemically.

20. C: Diazepam is a benzodiazepine drug that has several clinical indications. In prescribed doses, it can function as an anxiolytic, a short-duration anticonvulsant, a muscle relaxant, and an appetite stimulant. Diazepam does not, however, provide any analgesia when administered by itself and therefore must be used in conjunction with specific pain-relieving drugs, such as opioids, when used for anesthetic purposes.

21. C: Ultrasonography provides the earliest detection of pregnancy on day 20 of gestation in small animals. At this time the gestational sac should be readily visible.

22. C: It is always recommended to transfuse fresh whole blood immediately after collection so that the patient reaps the benefits of all the active components (coagulation factors, platelets, etc). If this is not possible, however, the blood may be transfused within the next 6-8 hours and still retain is effectiveness. After 8 hours, the blood will need to be refrigerated to preserve the blood components that are still useful (proteins, cells, Vitamin K dependent clotting factors). Platelets and other more "delicate" coagulation factors in the blood become ineffective over time and with refrigeration.

23. C: Bruising is a common sequela of intramuscular injections. Any bruised meat that is found at the time of slaughter will be either trimmed away, if possible, or thrown out all together, which results in a financial loss for the cattle rancher.

24. C: The transducer frequency is ultimately responsible for the resolution of the ultrasound image. As frequency increases, the wavelength decreases and shorter wavelengths produce better resolution and overall quality of the image.

25. C: Ventricular premature complexes (VPCs) occur as a result of an ectopic foci that discharge anywhere in the myocardial wall of the ventricle. The impulse is conducted cell-to-cell through the myocardium at a slow rate, versus more quickly through the intended Purkinje system, thereby producing an abnormally wide and bizarre QRS-T complex on ECG. VPCs are commonly seen with primary cardiac disease, secondary to trauma or systemic disease, or secondary to drug therapy. It is important to understand that they rarely cause any hemodynamic impairment unless they occur frequently, in which case they should be treated to prevent progression to more serious and potentially fatal arrhythmias such as ventricular tachycardia or ventricular fibrillation.

26. B: Obesity is the most common diet-related illness in pet hedgehogs and may occur as a result of overfeeding, lack of exercise, or high-fat diets. Obesity may lead to poor skin condition, hepatic lipidosis, respiratory and/or immune related disease, as well as skin fold dermatitis. It is therefore important to monitor the animal's weight frequently and to adjust the amount or type of food fed to the animal accordingly. Rickets and periodontal disease are other types of diet-related illness in hedgehogs that occur in unbalanced diets or diets that lack a hard consistency.

27. C: Acoustic shadowing is produced when soundwaves fail to travel through certain tissue like bone, or anomalies like bladder or gall stones. Since these soundwaves are completely attenuated, there is a shadow present directly posterior to these types of structures due to an absence of echoes.

28. D: Etomidate is a fast acting and short-lived induction agent that produces minimal cardiopulmonary effects, and is therefore the anesthetic of choice in patients with heart disease. Heart rate and rhythm, blood pressure, as well as respiratory rate are all maintained throughout anesthesia. Due to its short duration of action, etomidate is ideal to conduct brief studies such as examination and diagnostics on patients in extreme distress from cardiopulmonary disease that could easily die with any manipulation.

29. C: Crenation occurs when RBCs lose water through osmosis because the extracellular fluid is more concentrated (hypertonic) than the intracellular fluid (isotonic).
Hemolysis occurs when RBCs gain water through osmosis because the extracellular fluid is less concentrated (hypotonic) than the intracellular fluid.
Clumping of RBCs is termed autoagglutination and is usually indicative of immune-mediated hemolytic anemia.
RBCs that are clumped or stacked into a linear arrangement create a rouleaux formation (a normal finding in horses).

30. A:A nasogastric tube placed properly into the ventral meatus will feed easily into the esophagus and meet little resistance along the way, providing there are no obstructions such as tumors or foreign objects.
Excessive force during nasogastric intubation can damage the ethmoturbinates of the equine nasal passages, which will result in an exorbitant amount of bleeding. Force can also rupture the esophagus if there is a foreign body present.
An equine stomach should always be checked for gastric reflux before introducing any water or medication. If an abnormally large amount of ingesta is present in the stomach (this is usually indicated when ingesta flows freely out of the nasogastric tube), then the delivery of medication or water should be postponed until the stomach empties. This will reduce the risk of gastric overfilling and potential rupture.

31. D: Casts are formed by the slow movement of material in the renal tubules and are molded by the tubular lumen. Casts are comprised predominantly of a protein matrix that also contains substances that were present in the tubule when the cast was formed, such as hyaline, white or red blood cells, or epithelial cells. When present in large numbers, they indicate active renal disease. Few casts, however, may not be significant, especially if not found on repeat sediment exams.
Casts readily dissolve in alkaline urine, so it is imperative that urine samples be evaluated immediately before the urine chemistry changes.

32. C: Malignant melanoma is the most common oropharyngeal tumor in dogs and is usually located on the gingiva or on the buccal or labial mucosa. It may or may not be pigmented. Metastasis is very common with malignant melanoma (50% or more of cases), as is bone invasion (66% of cases), so preliminary diagnostics to determine stage of disease is recommended. Treatment usually involves a combination of surgical excision, radiation, immunotherapy, and/or chemotherapy. These treatments, however, still only afford a guarded prognosis.

33. D: Cutaneous larval migrans is a zoonotic disease in humans that is caused by the burrowing and migration of hookworm larvae intracutaneously, resulting in an intense dermatitis. Children who play in the dirt as well as people who are exposed to infected soil (gardeners, utility workers) are at risk of hookworm infection. These larvae migrate for long periods of time, and may penetrate into deeper tissues.
The zoonotic potential of many parasites necessitates the adoption of a comprehensive deworming program in any clinic. Technicians play a vital role in providing clients with vital information regarding these parasites so they can make informed decisions regarding the health of their pets and their families.

34. C: The periodontal ligament is composed of connective fibers that serve to anchor the tooth root to the alveolar bone. In addition to this function, the periodontal ligament also provides nutrients to the alveolar bone and cementum through a network of arterioles, and also serves as a "shock absorber" during mastication.

35. D: Dental polishing represents an integral part of the dental prophylaxis. Polishing decreases total tooth surface area by smoothing the enamel that was roughened and made irregular by the scaling process. By decreasing this surface area, polishing decreases the rate of plaque and calculus reattachment.

36. D: Mechanical scalers are an indispensable instrument during any prophylaxis and must be used properly to avoid accidental heat damage to the tooth surface. The amount of heat generated by the scaler can be reduced by using large amounts of water during the scaling process to cool the teeth, limiting the time spent on each tooth to only 5-10 seconds a piece, and only using the scaler at the speed that is recommended for the particular unit. In addition, it also helps not to use excessive force with the scaler, which can also create heat and further damage the enamel, possibly exposing the pulp.

37. B: Iris scissors are small, fine, delicate scissors that are reserved for precise surgeries, usually involving the eye. Spencer scissors are used to remove sutures. Mayo scissors are common in surgery for cutting dense, thick tissue. Metzenbaum scissors are also used in surgery for delicate tissue dissection.

38. B: Rochester-Carmalt forceps are large, crushing, hemostatic forceps that are used to secure tissue bundles containing blood vessels such as uterine stumps or ovarian pedicles.

39. D: Instruments are placed in surgical milk following ultrasonic cleaning to keep the instruments lubricated as well as to help prevent the formation of rust. It has no cleaning or sterilizing properties.

40. B: The carbon dioxide absorbent needs to be changed after 6-8 hours of use, or every 30 days regardless of how little it has been used. The absorbent serves to "capture" exhaled CO_2 and convert it to carbonate. If all the absorbent has been consumed, the patient will start to accumulate CO_2 in the bloodstream (hypercapnia), which leads to respiratory acidosis.

41. D: A half hitch knot is recommended because it not only allows for easy release in case of an emergency, but also alleviates direct pressure on the skin when it is applied over 2 areas of contact.

42. D: When a surgeon requests a drain during a surgical procedure, he/she is anticipating an accumulation of air (dead space) or fluid (ie, pus, serum, blood) in and/or around the surgical site. Procedures or conditions that warrant drain placement include abscesses, removal of large tumors that leave large gaps in muscle or tissue, limb amputation, or wounds that are difficult to clean completely. If drains are not utilized for these types of situations, the surgical site could swell or leak fluid, or continue to be infected, all of which can lead to suture dehiscence and the need for more surgery.

43. A: Hydrogen peroxide is a common foaming wound irrigant that should only be used once for the initial cleansing of a contaminated wound. If used repeatedly, hydrogen peroxide can damage the surrounding healthy tissue, which results in delayed wound healing.
Hydrogen peroxide does not possess any significant antimicrobial properties and thus should not be used solely for this purpose. It does, however, have a certain amount of effectiveness against spores.

44. B: Chlorhexidine and povidone-iodine scrubs share many properties, however only povidone-iodine scrub is inactivated by alcohol and organic matter such as blood or body fluids.

45. B: Electric heating pads are extremely dangerous when used to warm an animal and should never be used. They provide intense, focal areas of heat to which an unconscious animal cannot react, resulting in very painful and necrosing thermal burns.

46. B: Butorphanol should not be used in conjunction with fentanyl or any pure opioid agonist because it blocks the receptor (mu) in the brain to which the opioids bind to produce analgesia. Butorphanol is a mixed opioid agonist/antagonist meaning it stimulates certain receptors of the brain (kappa) to produce mild analgesia and moderate sedation, however it blocks the mu receptors, which are responsible for profound analgesia and mild sedation. So, when used together, a patient only receives the fleeting (45 minutes) analgesic effects of butorphanol versus the longer analgesic duration of the other pure opioid agonists, and is therefore experiencing pain most of the time.

47. A: Buprenorphine is an opioid analgesic in small animals that is used to control mild to moderate pain. Due to the unusual chemistry of the feline oral cavity, buprenorphine can be administered orally and still retain the same efficacy as an intramuscular or intravenous injection.

48. C: Glycopyrrolate is a preanesthetic anticholinergic that prevents or remedies the adverse effects (bradycardia, hypersalivation) of opioids, barbiturates, and dissociative anesthetics such as morphine, thiopental, and ketamine, respectively. As a parasympatholytic drug, glycopyrrolate also functions as a mydriatic, a bronchodilator as well as in inhibitor of intestinal motility. Because glycopyrrolate does not cross significantly through the blood-brain barrier, its effects on the central nervous system are less pronounced. It also should be noted that glycopyrrolate does not cross the placental barrier, which makes it an excellent preanesthetic drug for pregnant animals.

49. A: Stay sutures are an invaluable tool for isolating and elevating hollow organs that need to be incised, such as the bladder, intestine, or stomach. They are placed in the serosal surface of these organs on either side of the incision linearly and then secured with mosquito forceps. The organ is then gently elevated out of the abdominal cavity and placed over laparotomy pads, which will catch or reduce any spillage of urine or intestinal material that would otherwise contaminate the surgical area. They allow for better visualization and control over the surgical site.

50. B: Enalapril is an angiotensin-converting enzyme inhibitor and functions to reduce the workload on a diseased heart by promoting vasodilation.

Diuretics are substances that promote urine secretion, usually through a mechanism that enhances the excretion of sodium and water in the renal tubules. They are most commonly used to treat edema that occurs as a result of congestive heart failure, liver failure, or neuronal edema from head trauma. For example, mannitol is an osmotic diuretic that has a low molecular weight and is freely filtered by the kidneys. Its presence in the kidney will draw water and sodium into the tubules, thereby increasing urine flow. It is used primary in cases of cerebral edema.

Furosemide is a drug that inhibits sodium chloride reabsorption in the ascending loop of Henle, again serving to increase urine flow. This drug is commonly used for congestive heart failure.

Spironolactone is a drug that blocks the effects of the hormone aldosterone, a hormone that would ordinarily allow for sodium reabsorption in the renal tubules.

Secret Key #1 - Time is Your Greatest Enemy

Pace Yourself

Wear a watch. At the beginning of the test, check the time (or start a chronometer on your watch to count the minutes), and check the time after every few questions to make sure you are "on schedule."

If you are forced to speed up, do it efficiently. Usually one or more answer choices can be eliminated without too much difficulty. Above all, don't panic. Don't speed up and just begin guessing at random choices. By pacing yourself, and continually monitoring your progress against your watch, you will always know exactly how far ahead or behind you are with your available time. If you find that you are one minute behind on the test, don't skip one question without spending any time on it, just to catch back up. Take 15 fewer seconds on the next four questions, and after four questions you'll have caught back up. Once you catch back up, you can continue working each problem at your normal pace.

Furthermore, don't dwell on the problems that you were rushed on. If a problem was taking up too much time and you made a hurried guess, it must be difficult. The difficult questions are the ones you are most likely to miss anyway, so it isn't a big loss. It is better to end with more time than you need than to run out of time.

Lastly, sometimes it is beneficial to slow down if you are constantly getting ahead of time. You are always more likely to catch a careless mistake by working more slowly than quickly, and among very high-scoring test takers (those who are likely to have lots of time left over), careless errors affect the score more than mastery of material.

Secret Key #2 - Guessing is not Guesswork

You probably know that guessing is a good idea - unlike other standardized tests, there is no penalty for getting a wrong answer. Even if you have no idea about a question, you still have a 20-25% chance of getting it right.

Most test takers do not understand the impact that proper guessing can have on their score. Unless you score extremely high, guessing will significantly contribute to your final score.

Monkeys Take the Test

What most test takers don't realize is that to insure that 20-25% chance, you have to guess randomly. If you put 20 monkeys in a room to take this test, assuming they answered once per question and behaved themselves, on average they would get 20-25% of the questions correct. Put 20 test takers in the room, and the average will be much lower among guessed questions. Why?
1. The test writers intentionally writes deceptive answer choices that "look" right. A test taker has no idea about a question, so picks the "best looking" answer, which is often wrong. The monkey has no idea what looks good and what doesn't, so will consistently be lucky about 20-25% of the time.
2. Test takers will eliminate answer choices from the guessing pool based on a hunch or intuition. Simple but correct answers often get excluded, leaving a 0% chance of being correct. The monkey has no clue, and often gets lucky with the best choice.

This is why the process of elimination endorsed by most test courses is flawed and detrimental to your performance- test takers don't guess, they make an ignorant stab in the dark that is usually worse than random.

$5 Challenge

Let me introduce one of the most valuable ideas of this course- the $5 challenge:

You only mark your "best guess" if you are willing to bet $5 on it.
You only eliminate choices from guessing if you are willing to bet $5 on it.

Why $5? Five dollars is an amount of money that is small yet not insignificant, and can really add up fast (20 questions could cost you $100). Likewise, each answer choice on one question of the test will have a small impact on your overall score, but it can really add up to a lot of points in the end.

The process of elimination IS valuable. The following shows your chance of guessing it right:

If you eliminate wrong answer choices until only this many remain:	1	2	3
Chance of getting it correct:	100%	50%	33%

However, if you accidentally eliminate the right answer or go on a hunch for an incorrect answer, your chances drop dramatically: to 0%. By guessing among all the answer choices, you are GUARANTEED to have a shot at the right answer.

That's why the $5 test is so valuable- if you give up the advantage and safety of a pure guess, it had better be worth the risk.

What we still haven't covered is how to be sure that whatever guess you make is truly random. Here's the easiest way:

Always pick the first answer choice among those remaining.

Such a technique means that you have decided, **before you see a single test question**, exactly how you are going to guess- and since the order of choices tells you nothing about which one is correct, this guessing technique is perfectly random.

This section is not meant to scare you away from making educated guesses or eliminating choices- you just need to define when a choice is worth eliminating. The $5 test, along with a pre-defined random guessing strategy, is the best way to make sure you reap all of the benefits of guessing.

Secret Key #3 - Practice Smarter, Not Harder

Many test takers delay the test preparation process because they dread the awful amounts of practice time they think necessary to succeed on the test. We have refined an effective method that will take you only a fraction of the time.

There are a number of "obstacles" in your way to succeed. Among these are answering questions, finishing in time, and mastering test-taking strategies. All must be executed on the day of the test at peak performance, or your score will suffer. The test is a mental marathon that has a large impact on your future.

Just like a marathon runner, it is important to work your way up to the full challenge. So first you just worry about questions, and then time, and finally strategy:

Success Strategy

1. Find a good source for practice tests.
2. If you are willing to make a larger time investment, consider using more than one study guide- often the different approaches of multiple authors will help you "get" difficult concepts.

3. Take a practice test with no time constraints, with all study helps "open book." Take your time with questions and focus on applying strategies.
4. Take a practice test with time constraints, with all guides "open book."
5. Take a final practice test with no open material and time limits

If you have time to take more practice tests, just repeat step 5. By gradually exposing yourself to the full rigors of the test environment, you will condition your mind to the stress of test day and maximize your success.

Secret Key #4 - Prepare, Don't Procrastinate

Let me state an obvious fact: if you take the test three times, you will get three different scores. This is due to the way you feel on test day, the level of preparedness you have, and, despite the test writers' claims to the contrary, some tests WILL be easier for you than others.

Since your future depends so much on your score, you should maximize your chances of success. In order to maximize the likelihood of success, you've got to prepare in advance. This means taking practice tests and spending time learning the information and test taking strategies you will need to succeed.

Never take the test as a "practice" test, expecting that you can just take it again if you need to. Feel free to take sample tests on your own, but when you go to take the official test, be prepared, be focused, and do your best the first time!

Secret Key #5 - Test Yourself

Everyone knows that time is money. There is no need to spend too much of your time or too little of your time preparing for the test. You should only spend as much of your precious time preparing as is necessary for you to get the score you need.

Once you have taken a practice test under real conditions of time constraints, then you will know if you are ready for the test or not.

If you have scored extremely high the first time that you take the practice test, then there is not much point in spending countless hours studying. You are already there.

Benchmark your abilities by retaking practice tests and seeing how much you have improved. Once you score high enough to guarantee success, then you are ready.

If you have scored well below where you need, then knuckle down and begin studying in earnest. Check your improvement regularly through the use of practice tests under real conditions. Above all, don't worry, panic, or give up. The key is perseverance!

Then, when you go to take the test, remain confident and remember how well you did on the practice tests. If you can score high enough on a practice test, then you can do the same on the real thing.

The most important thing you can do is to ignore your fears and jump into the test immediately- do not be overwhelmed by any strange-sounding terms. You have to jump into the test like jumping into a pool- all at once is the easiest way.

Make Predictions

As you read and understand the question, try to guess what the answer will be. Remember that several of the answer choices are wrong, and once you begin reading them, your mind will immediately become cluttered with answer choices designed to throw you off. Your mind is typically the most focused immediately after you have read the question and digested its contents. If you can, try to predict what the correct answer will be. You may be surprised at what you can predict.

Quickly scan the choices and see if your prediction is in the listed answer choices. If it is, then you can be quite confident that you have the right answer. It still won't hurt to check the other answer choices, but most of the time, you've got it!

Answer the Question

It may seem obvious to only pick answer choices that answer the question, but the test writers can create some excellent answer choices that are wrong. Don't pick an answer just because it sounds right, or you believe it to be true. It MUST answer the question. Once you've made your selection, always go back and check it against the question and make sure that you didn't misread the question, and the answer choice does answer the question posed.

Benchmark

After you read the first answer choice, decide if you think it sounds correct or not. If it doesn't, move on to the next answer choice. If it does, mentally mark that answer choice. This doesn't mean that you've definitely selected it as your answer choice, it just means that it's the best you've seen thus far. Go ahead and read the next choice. If the next choice is worse than the one you've already selected, keep going to the next answer choice. If the next choice is better than the choice you've already selected, mentally mark the new answer choice as your best guess.

The first answer choice that you select becomes your standard. Every other answer choice must be benchmarked against that standard. That choice is correct until proven otherwise by another answer choice beating it out. Once you've decided that no other answer choice seems as good, do one final check to ensure that your answer choice answers the question posed.

Valid Information

Don't discount any of the information provided in the question. Every piece of information may be necessary to determine the correct answer. None of the information in the question is there to throw you off (while the answer choices will certainly have information to throw you off). If two seemingly unrelated topics are discussed, don't ignore either. You can be confident there is a relationship, or it wouldn't be included in the question, and you are probably going to have to determine what is that relationship to find the answer.

Avoid "Fact Traps"

Don't get distracted by a choice that is factually true. Your search is for the answer that answers the question. Stay focused and don't fall for an answer that is true but incorrect. Always go back to the question and make sure you're choosing an answer that actually answers the question and is not just a true statement. An answer can be factually correct, but it MUST answer the question asked. Additionally, two answers can both be seemingly correct, so be sure to read all of the answer choices, and make sure that you get the one that BEST answers the question.

Milk the Question

Some of the questions may throw you completely off. They might deal with a subject you have not been exposed to, or one that you haven't reviewed in years. While your lack of knowledge about the subject will be a hindrance, the question itself can give you many clues that will help you find the correct answer. Read the question carefully and look for clues. Watch particularly for adjectives and nouns describing difficult terms or words that you don't recognize. Regardless of if you completely understand a word or not, replacing it with a synonym either provided or one you more familiar with may help you to understand what the questions are asking. Rather than wracking your mind about specific detailed information concerning a difficult term or word, try to use mental substitutes that are easier to understand.

The Trap of Familiarity

Don't just choose a word because you recognize it. On difficult questions, you may not recognize a number of words in the answer choices. The test writers don't put "make-believe" words on the test; so don't think that just because you only recognize all the words in one answer choice means that answer choice must be correct. If you only recognize words in one answer choice, then focus on that one. Is it correct? Try your best to determine if it is correct. If it is, that is great, but if it doesn't, eliminate it. Each word and answer choice you eliminate increases your chances of getting the question correct, even if you then have to guess among the unfamiliar choices.

Eliminate Answers

Eliminate choices as soon as you realize they are wrong. But be careful! Make sure you consider all of the possible answer choices. Just because one appears right, doesn't mean that the next one won't be even better! The test writers will usually put more than one good answer choice for every question, so read all of them. Don't worry if you are stuck between two that seem right. By getting down to just two remaining possible choices, your odds are now 50/50. Rather than wasting too much time, play the odds. You are guessing, but guessing wisely, because you've been able to knock out some of the answer choices that you know are wrong. If you are eliminating choices and realize that the last answer choice you are left with is also obviously wrong, don't panic. Start over and consider each choice again. There may easily be something that you missed the first time and will realize on the second pass.

Tough Questions

If you are stumped on a problem or it appears too hard or too difficult, don't waste time. Move on! Remember though, if you can quickly check for obviously incorrect answer choices, your chances of guessing correctly are greatly improved. Before you completely give up, at least try to knock out a couple of possible answers. Eliminate what you can and then guess at the remaining answer choices before moving on.

Brainstorm

If you get stuck on a difficult question, spend a few seconds quickly brainstorming. Run through the complete list of possible answer choices. Look at each choice and ask yourself, "Could this answer the question satisfactorily?" Go through each answer choice and consider it independently of the other. By systematically going through all possibilities, you may find something that you would otherwise overlook. Remember that when you get stuck, it's important to try to keep moving.

Read Carefully

Understand the problem. Read the question and answer choices carefully. Don't miss the question because you misread the terms. You have plenty of time to read each question thoroughly and make sure you understand what is being asked. Yet a happy medium must be attained, so don't waste too much time. You must read carefully, but efficiently.

Face Value

When in doubt, use common sense. Always accept the situation in the problem at face value. Don't read too much into it. These problems will not require you to make huge leaps of logic. The test writers aren't trying

Copyright © Mometrix Media. You have been licensed one copy of this document for personal use only.
Any other reproduction or redistribution is strictly prohibited. All rights reserved.

to throw you off with a cheap trick. If you have to go beyond creativity and make a leap of logic in order to have an answer choice answer the question, then you should look at the other answer choices. Don't overcomplicate the problem by creating theoretical relationships or explanations that will warp time or space. These are normal problems rooted in reality. It's just that the applicable relationship or explanation may not be readily apparent and you have to figure things out. Use your common sense to interpret anything that isn't clear.

Prefixes

If you're having trouble with a word in the question or answer choices, try dissecting it. Take advantage of every clue that the word might include. Prefixes and suffixes can be a huge help. Usually they allow you to determine a basic meaning. Pre- means before, post- means after, pro - is positive, de- is negative. From these prefixes and suffixes, you can get an idea of the general meaning of the word and try to put it into context. Beware though of any traps. Just because con is the opposite of pro, doesn't necessarily mean congress is the opposite of progress!

Hedge Phrases

Watch out for critical "hedge" phrases, such as likely, may, can, will often, sometimes, often, almost, mostly, usually, generally, rarely, sometimes. Question writers insert these hedge phrases to cover every possibility. Often an answer choice will be wrong simply because it leaves no room for exception. Avoid answer choices that have definitive words like "exactly," and "always".

Switchback Words

Stay alert for "switchbacks". These are the words and phrases frequently used to alert you to shifts in thought. The most common switchback word is "but". Others include although, however, nevertheless, on the other hand, even though, while, in spite of, despite, regardless of.

New Information

Correct answer choices will rarely have completely new information included. Answer choices typically are straightforward reflections of the material asked about and will directly relate to the question. If a new piece of information is included in an answer choice that doesn't even seem to relate to the topic being asked about, then that answer choice is likely incorrect. All of the information needed to answer the question is usually provided for you, and so you should not have to make guesses that are unsupported or choose answer choices that require unknown information that cannot be reasoned on its own.

Time Management

On technical questions, don't get lost on the technical terms. Don't spend too much time on any one question. If you don't know what a term means, then since you don't have a dictionary, odds are you aren't going to get much further. You should immediately recognize terms as whether or not you know them. If you don't, work with the other clues that you have, the other answer choices and terms provided, but don't waste too much time trying to figure out a difficult term.

Contextual Clues

Look for contextual clues. An answer can be right but not correct. The contextual clues will help you find the answer that is most right and is correct. Understand the context in which a phrase or statement is made. This will help you make important distinctions.

Don't Panic

Panicking will not answer any questions for you. Therefore, it isn't helpful. When you first see the question, if your mind goes blank, take a deep breath. Force yourself to mechanically go through the steps of solving the problem and using the strategies you've learned.

Pace Yourself

Don't get clock fever. It's easy to be overwhelmed when you're looking at a page full of questions, your mind is full of random thoughts and feeling confused, and the clock is ticking down faster than you would like. Calm down and maintain the pace that you have set for yourself. As long as you are on track by monitoring your pace, you are guaranteed to have enough time for yourself. When you get to the last few minutes of the test, it may seem like you won't have enough time left, but if you only have as many questions as you should have left at that point, then you're right on track!

Answer Selection

The best way to pick an answer choice is to eliminate all of those that are wrong, until only one is left and confirm that is the correct answer. Sometimes though, an answer choice may immediately look right. Be careful! Take a second to make sure that the other choices are not equally obvious. Don't make a hasty mistake. There are only two times that you should stop before checking other answers. First is when you are positive that the answer choice you have selected is correct. Second is when time is almost out and you have to make a quick guess!

Check Your Work

Since you will probably not know every term listed and the answer to every question, it is important that you get credit for the ones that you do know. Don't miss any questions through careless mistakes. If at all possible, try to take a second to look back over your answer selection and make sure you've selected the correct answer choice and haven't made a costly careless mistake (such as marking an answer choice that you didn't mean to mark). This quick double check should more than pay for itself in caught mistakes for the time it costs.

Beware of Directly Quoted Answers

Sometimes an answer choice will repeat word for word a portion of the question or reference section. However, beware of such exact duplication – it may be a trap! More than likely, the correct choice will paraphrase or summarize a point, rather than being exactly the same wording.

Slang

Scientific sounding answers are better than slang ones. An answer choice that begins "To compare the outcomes..." is much more likely to be correct than one that begins "Because some people insisted..."

Extreme Statements

Avoid wild answers that throw out highly controversial ideas that are proclaimed as established fact. An answer choice that states the "process should be used in certain situations, if..." is much more likely to be correct than one that states the "process should be discontinued completely." The first is a calm rational statement and doesn't even make a definitive, uncompromising stance, using a hedge word "if" to provide wiggle room, whereas the second choice is a radical idea and far more extreme.

Answer Choice Families

When you have two or more answer choices that are direct opposites or parallels, one of them is usually the correct answer. For instance, if one answer choice states "x increases" and another answer choice states "x decreases" or "y increases," then those two or three answer choices are very similar in construction and fall into the same family of answer choices. A family of answer choices is when two or three answer choices are very similar in construction, and yet often have a directly opposite meaning. Usually the correct answer choice will be in that family of answer choices. The "odd man out" or answer choice that doesn't seem to fit the parallel construction of the other answer choices is more likely to be incorrect.

Special Report: Additional Bonus Material

Due to our efforts to try to keep this book to a manageable length, we've created a link that will give you access to all of your additional bonus material.

Please visit http://www.mometrix.com/bonus948/vtne to access the information.